HOW TO HELP
SOMEONE WITH
DEMENTIA

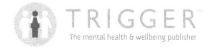

TRIGGER
The mental health & wellbeing publisher

ABOUT THE AUTHORS

Dr Michelle Hamill is a consultant clinical psychologist who has worked in the NHS for over 15 years in the field of older adult mental health, memory clinics and dementia care. She has a particular interest in relationship-based psychological therapies.

Dr Martina McCarthy is a clinical psychologist with over 10 years' experience in the NHS, specializing in memory clinic work and strength-based psychological therapies for people with dementia and older adults, along with family work.

Michelle and Martina are both from Ireland. Their clinical work has been informed and shaped by personal experiences of dementia care.

I've had the privilege of working with Dr Hamill and Dr McCarthy for many years and have seen the positive impact their work has had. They – and the carers and people with dementia who have helped produce this book – have distilled their positive, strengths-based approach and an absolute wealth of learning into a wonderfully accessible, informative and generous guide to caring for a person with dementia and for oneself as a carer. Despite 25 years of experience with dementia, I have learned plenty here to take back into clinical practice. How to Help Someone with Dementia synthesizes the very best available practical advice and evidence on the subject. I highly recommend this book to everyone involved in dementia care.

Dr Juliette Brown, Consultant Psychiatrist, East London NHS Foundation Trust, Honorary Clinical Senior Lecturer in the Centre for Psychiatry, Wolfson Institute of Preventative Medicine, Queen Mary University London (QMUL)

HOW TO HELP SOMEONE WITH DEMENTIA

A Practical Guide to Caring for Your
Loved One and Yourself

Dr Michelle Hamill and Dr Martina McCarthy

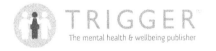

TRIGGER

The mental health & wellbeing publisher

This edition published in 2023 by Trigger Publishing
An imprint of Shaw Callaghan Ltd

UK Office
The Stanley Building
7 Pancras Square
Kings Cross
London N1C 4AG

US Office
On Point Executive Center, Inc
3030 N Rocky Point Drive W
Suite 150
Tampa, FL 33607
www.triggerhub.org

A CIP catalogue record for this book is available upon request from the British Library
ISBN: 978-1-83796-260-0
Ebook ISBN: 978-1-83796-261-7

Typeset by Lapiz Digital Services

This book is dedicated to every carer and person with dementia who has taught us in our work, and for others around the world. Your bravery, courage, compassion, and your dedication to living well with dementia, makes the world a better place.

To Emily and Reilly, Mum and Dad – my biggest cheerleaders.
Michelle

To my grandmother Hannah who lived so well with dementia and was enabled to do so by my wonderful parents, Kathleen and Joseph.
Martina

A big thank you to Patrisha David, Shirley Drake and Edna Medland for generously sharing their stories, which enabled us to reach new insights in writing this book.

In memory of Eileen Florence McDermott and Robert 'Bob' Medland.

.

CONTENTS

INTRODUCTION

"Changing our approach can produce more wellbeing for people living with dementia than any pill that is available today or is likely to be available in the foreseeable future."

Dr Allen Power, Geriatrician and board member of
US Dementia Action Alliance

There can be a lot of fear and understandable worry when a loved one receives a diagnosis of dementia. The aim of this book is to help you feel less alone in your journey, drawing from the experiences and voices of people we have worked with. This includes carers, who have long supported loved ones with dementia, as well as people living with dementia themselves. As accredited clinical psychologists working in dementia care, we aim to provide evidence-based information and advice to help you do the best for your loved one, whilst also looking after yourself.

Everyone's experience and situation is unique, but we hope to provide insights and ideas to improve quality of life for both you and your loved one. We understand that whilst the stigma of dementia can be powerful, it should not restrict anyone from finding meaning and purpose in life. We believe that a person-centred understanding of dementia can help to acknowledge the challenges of the condition, whilst valuing the uniqueness of each individual and enabling them to live well and with dignity.

We will present ideas and strategies that have helped the people we have worked with over many years. We draw on a wide range of psychological approaches, based on contemporary research, to tailor our work to meet different individual and carer needs. Our work is informed by international experts in their respective fields of dementia care and emotional wellbeing, alongside the real experts – the people with dementia and their carers, who inspire and teach us.

By reading the book you will:

- Understand dementia and the associated symptoms and behaviours that can arise.
- Develop skills of person-centred care to improve your loved one's quality of life.
- Learn the importance of looking after yourself.
- Learn how to communicate more effectively with your loved one.
- Troubleshoot some of the more common problems that arise.

A NOTE ABOUT TERMINOLOGY

There is much debate regarding appropriate terminology when describing family and friends who take on a caring role, as well as to describe a person with dementia. We have chosen to use 'loved one' to describe the person with dementia who is being supported. Our rationale is summarized in the 2019 World Alzheimer Report by Elder Jerry Otowadjiwan, who reminds us that "the person with dementia, who is being cared for, needs a lot of love". He urges the use of 'loved one' to refer to the person with dementia, so that we remember that they are loved and to serve as a reminder of how care providers should be treating and respecting the person with dementia.

You may not think of yourself as a 'carer', particularly if the person with dementia is your parent, partner or close friend, and the term may sit uncomfortably if the role has been taken on without a conscious decision or choice. However, as time goes by, your loved one will require increasing levels of care and support and, as such, we feel that 'carer' is an appropriate term to describe your role.

HOW THIS BOOK WORKS

This book is best read chronologically to help you and your loved one along the dementia journey. However, each chapter can also be read as a standalone chapter, which you can dip in and out of depending on your needs and where you are at any given time in this experience. In each chapter you will see exercises to help you to reflect on yourself and your approach, as well as 'how to help' boxes with plenty of strategies to support your loved one.

Chapter 1 looks at the narratives around dementia and how it can be viewed differently depending on these, and introduces the principles of person-centred care, a values-based approach that honours every person with dementia, with dignity and relationships at its core.

Chapter 2 examines dementia in more detail. Despite common features, there is no universal path to follow as each person's condition progresses differently depending on their unique biology, life context, and social circumstances.

Chapter 3 explores coming to terms with the diagnosis and considers the values that will help to guide your actions as a carer.

Chapter 4 focuses on ideas for enhancing your loved one's wellbeing and quality of life.

Chapter 5 looks at *your* health and wellbeing, and how to develop resilience in the face of challenges.

Chapter 6 offers advice and strategies to improve communication between you and your loved one, from the early to the more advanced stages of dementia.

Chapter 7 examines strategies for helping with the behavioural and psychological symptoms associated with dementia that can be challenging.

Chapter 8 looks at transitions around formal care arrangements and considerations around end-of-life care.

THE LIVED EXPERIENCE

Throughout the book, you will hear from the lived experience of a person with dementia, as well as carers we have worked with. We share anonymized accounts of our clinical experiences too – stories of families and couples we have worked directly with throughout the years. With permission, Patrisha, Shirley and Edna impart their knowledge and expertise about many issues encountered during their dementia journeys.

Patrisha is a 64-year-old woman who is living with a rare dementia associated with Progressive Supranuclear Palsy.

Shirley cared for her mother Eileen with Alzheimer's dementia for many years, both in the community and in a care home. Eileen died aged 96 during the writing of this book.

Edna looked after her husband Bob with vascular dementia at home until poor health resulted in a care home stay. Bob died at the age of 89.

Their voices form the heart of this book. By contributing, Patrisha, Shirley and Edna's hope is for their stories to help others; we feel strongly that they do. Their lived experiences demonstrate the reality and sadness that comes with dementia and caring alongside creativity, strength, compassion, and hope. We hope that the energy we have gained from Patrisha, Shirley and Edna reaches you too and helps to sustain you in the journey ahead.

The ideas and strategies in this book can help you to maintain a good quality of life and derive meaning and purpose from this experience. Bearing witness to the changes that are possible, regardless of the stage of dementia, and the extent of people's resilience within our work, really is a privilege. Throughout this book, we want to convey the lived experience of dementia and help to sustain you as a carer. We want to show you what is possible and how to live well with dementia. We have done so in a collaborative way, with privacy and dignity at the heart of this sharing. The stories of Patrisha, Edna and Shirley, amongst others, bring a realism as well as a celebration of rich, important, and meaningful lives. Despite the loss of abilities that come with dementia, this book will support you to see that your loved one remains a unique individual with a rich history, important relationships, achievements, disappointments, and interests; someone who can continue to contribute to your relationship, right up until the end.

Above all, this book is about getting you ready to collaborate with your loved one; not to just 'do things' for them. Together, we can work to challenge the stigma of dementia and build a more humane and inclusive world for everyone to live in.

CHAPTER 1

SETTING THE SCENE

"People with dementia may have something important to teach the rest of humankind. If we make the venture one of genuine and open engagement, we will learn a great deal about ourselves."

Professor Tom Kitwood, Professor of Psychogerontology and founder of Bradford Dementia Group

Have you ever felt as if caring for your loved one is like a rollercoaster of ups and downs? Perhaps you have felt despondent and overwhelmed one day, then satisfied and content the next? Maybe you feel you have grasped 'dementia', only for your loved one to do something that makes you feel like a total novice? If so, then you are not alone. Caring for someone with dementia is often compared to marathon training: at times it can be overwhelming and painful, and you might feel like giving up, but learning to pace yourself through self-care and finding purpose, even in the face of the most difficult times, will ensure that you can go the distance. Everyone's caring journey will differ but there are core skills and strategies that you can learn to help you along the way, irrespective of the stage of your loved one's dementia.

BUILDING STRENGTH THROUGH TELLING A DIFFERENT STORY

"Stories bring awareness to the type of person you are – the whole of me. I want to be able to connect to the positive about myself through stories."
Patrisha

The ability to tell stories is a fundamental part of what makes us human and shapes our thinking. Much of our knowledge and thinking is organized in story form, and therefore stories offer us a means to make sense of the present, look to the future, and plan and create meaning in our lives. The words we use and the stories that we tell ourselves shape our experiences, mood, and wellbeing. Words are incredibly powerful and those we choose set the tone for our lives – they can be hopeful and encouraging or restrictive and damaging. This is no more evident than in the language used to describe dementia: it is often labelled as a 'living death', where the person becomes a 'shell of their former selves'. Discussions about dementia often focus on the social, health and economic burden; we see attempts to 'attack' or 'combat' the disease through medical cures, and terms such as 'epidemic', 'crisis' and 'plague' to describe its prevalence. Dementia discourses around the world often frame dementia solely in terms of atrophied brains, personal tragedy, and negativity, overlooking the uniqueness of the person and their life experiences.

> *"People with dementia are still human beings and should be recognized and allowed to enjoy every minute of their life the best they can! We have an opportunity to significantly improve the lives of people affected by dementia and memory loss in our community."*
> *Shirley*

Shirley frames all of us as 'enablers', which is a message of hope and opportunity. Working with people like Patrisha, Shirley and Edna inspires us to offer a different approach to the narrow and unhelpful focus on treating the biology of the disease, which has done little to truly improve the lives of those living with dementia. Society further disables people with dementia through prejudicial attitudes, poorly adapted environments and public policies that make life harder.

Experiencing dementia is hard enough but it is made so much harder by the stigma surrounding it, which has far more destructive consequences than the disease process itself, compromising people's self-worth and resulting in isolation and shame.

> *"There is generally a poor understanding and poor awareness about dementia in society. I am tired of assumptions being made about me. I am more than a brain and I have lived a rich and interesting life. I am more than dementia."*
> *Patrisha*

How can we address the negative narratives or stories around dementia? How can we try to undo the fear that is internalized and believed by the person with dementia and their families? As psychologists, we are often placed to help to alleviate the hurt and upset. This can prove difficult given dementia care is typically subject to problem-focused accounts. Whilst we cannot deny the challenges that can arise when caring for a loved one with dementia, we will also talk about hope. Yes, hope!

> *"I am hopeful for myself. I have a natural drive and determination. I want to be positive and to have a quality of life. I want to have fun and laughter. I want to be able to do things for myself for as long as possible. Being social and staying connected to family*

*and friends is important to me. I want people to know this so
they can help me achieve my wishes."*
Patrisha

It is often the problem story that dominates the life of the person with dementia and their family. However, focusing solely on difficulties reduces the opportunities for affirmative action. Whilst finding alternative meanings may be difficult for individuals as their dementia progresses, the people within their circle of support can help. Even as brain function declines, the stories and the person's identity remain held by those around them.

CHANGING THE NARRATIVE

We will show you how to create more strength-based stories that honour your unique life experience, where dementia plays a part but is far from the whole story. How do we do this? We will help you to focus on what is within your control, learning to adapt to the changes dementia brings and use your values to guide you, and with various adjustments support you both, right until the end stages. The nature of progression in dementia is hugely variable. It is a very individual experience and there is no one set path to follow. Although it is natural to jump ahead, imagining the end stages, this will inevitably result in your mind getting caught up in the worst-case scenarios. The reality is no one can predict what will happen in the future, yet we often spend a considerable amount of time preoccupied and trying to control it. We will be encouraging you to focus on where you and your loved one are at currently. Being in the moment and being together is what really counts. If this is difficult for your loved one, you may help to fill in the gaps. We will help you to move toward hope, where improvements in health and wellbeing are possible.

"Being in the moment and being together is what really counts."

We feel very privileged to work with you and to empower your loved one to consider your personal stories of strength, hope and empowerment. Despite the complications and unpredictable nature of dementia, you may surprise yourself with strength and reserve you never knew you had. There are rewards to be found in improving the wellbeing of a loved one, which can offer balance in the face of pain. This is what we have witnessed and experienced: love, joy, and a sense of deep connection, through tears, despair, frustrations, and laughter. Looking beyond the dementia – seeing your loved one as person – will sustain and nurture you both in this journey.

OUR CLINICAL AND THEORETICAL APPROACH

Within our clinical practice, we draw extensively on a variety of evidence-based psychological approaches, including:

- Cognitive Analytic Therapy (CAT)
- Acceptance and Commitment Therapy (ACT)
- Compassion Focused Therapy (CFT)
- Narrative Therapy (NT)
- Cognitive Behavioural Therapy (CBT)
- Systemic Therapy

This means that we can tailor our approaches to different individuals' and familys' needs and preferences to improve mental health and wellbeing. Whilst each of these therapeutic approaches differs, they all have at their core a focus on developing non-judgemental, compassionate self-awareness and learning how to reduce distress and better manage difficult thoughts, feelings, and physical sensations through active change. At the heart of these approaches lie the principles of person-centred care.

PERSON-CENTRED CARE: CARE FIT FOR VIPS

Person-centred care offers an alternative approach to dementia care and contrasts with traditional medical models, which focus predominantly on illness and disease. Person-centred care tells a different story about dementia. It offers a values-based approach that honours every person with dementia, with dignity and relationships at its core. Person-centred care takes the view that people with dementia are unique individuals whose life experiences and preferences must be always considered, whilst delivering quality care. This approach was first developed in the 1980s by British psychologist, Tom Kitwood. He spoke about a 'malignant social psychology', which means that in an unintentional way, social and interpersonal processes break down when people with dementia are categorized and deemed no longer to be individuals; easily done when focusing on a brain or diagnosis. Kitwood went on to define what is known as 'personhood', which is a status given to a human being by others and in the context of relationships.[1] It involves recognition, respect, and trust. Part of this is recognizing your loved one as a person with their own sense of self, with different roles in life: past and present.

> "I'm a 64-year-old retired nurse living with a rare dementia called Progressive Supranuclear Palsy. My identity has not changed since developing dementia. Nor has my past changed. Our behaviours and habits may change, but not our lives. Please consider what

is happening around us. Have perspective. Show us respect, dignity, and privacy."
Patrisha

Defining your loved one solely by dementia risks overlooking their deep need for emotional connection, purpose, and meaningful engagement, which persists right until the end of life. As Patrisha's experience shows us, personhood honours and celebrates personality, difference, and individuality. She was a highly accomplished nurse who, up until recently, travelled the world. Having met lots of people and having had lots of interesting experiences, she wants her rich life honoured and maintained. Person-centred care not only compensates for what people with dementia cannot do, but helps to facilitate their interests, pleasure and the use of abilities that remain intact.[2] Person-centred care puts your loved one's individual interests, background and needs first. It ensures that care is designed around them, rather than taking a one-size- fits-all approach.

> "Person-centred care puts your loved one's individual interests, background and needs first."

Looking at your loved one's uniqueness requires the ability to recognize the differences between us all. Let's consider all that makes us different. Social GRRAACCEESS, a model developed by British family-and-systemic psychotherapist John Burnham,[3] is a concise way to remind us about the aspects of difference within our personal and social identities along with beliefs, power, and lifestyle. Below are those factors that make us different:

- Gender
- Race
- Religion
- Age
- Ability
- Class
- Culture
- Education
- Ethnicity
- Sexuality
- Spirituality

This is a neat way to help broaden our views and allows us to consider wider contextual issues and their influences. Remember what Patrisha said. At times, it will be important to pay attention to areas of difference in our relationships, which can affect behaviours. Changes in power and control will lead to differences in your relationship with your loved one. Knowing these different parts allows you to explore more fully the influence of these particular aspects on the lives of you and your loved one. These factors may have a dominant presence or, alternatively, may be invisible or unnoticed.

> "A person-centred approach ensures your loved one's voice is heard, even when language starts to break down."

One of the central components of person-centred care is to promote and enable people to maintain their status as human beings first and foremost, despite the various challenges associated with dementia. Having a sense of agency and control, where dignity and privacy are respected, is closely related to independence, and needs to be carefully negotiated as dementia progresses. Being aware of power is important as power differentials permeate everything that we do, often resulting in struggles and upset. Adopting a person-centred approach ensures your loved one's voice is heard, even when language starts to break down. As you can see, this approach is not medicalized. Instead, it brings our attention to other essential factors in dementia care; those that surround the person in a more social and relational way. It is these factors that will offer you opportunities to focus your efforts, improve your loved one's wellbeing and bring meaning to the caring role.

VIPS CARE

Professor Dawn Brooker, a British clinical psychologist, has further defined the essential elements of person-centred care in her VIPS model.[4] VIPS is a handy acronym as many will understand its use for 'Very Important Persons'. VIPS breaks person-centred care into manageable parts (which are covered in each chapter throughout this book), acting as a guide for you in caring for your loved one. We suggest that you spend some time thinking about Professor Brooker's questions and reflections below. We understand that it is not always easy to follow these principles. Coming back to them, time and time again, will help you feel reassured that you are doing what you can to support your loved one.

V = Values people: People with dementia and their carers both need to be valued, and their rights respected and promoted. As you care for your loved one, consider: 'Do my actions value and honour my loved one as they live with dementia?'

I = Individual's needs: People with dementia need to be treated as individuals, with their background, personality, physical and mental health needs, social connections and financial conditions all considered. The care being provided needs to be adapted accordingly. Consider: 'Do I recognize the individual uniqueness of my loved one?'

P = Perspective of your loved one: It is important to look at the world from the perspective of your loved one, considering their individual needs and life circumstances. Ask yourself, 'Do I make a serious attempt to see my actions from their perspective or standpoint?'

S = Supportive social psychology: Humans are social creatures and maintaining social and personal relationships and interactions are essential to your loved one's wellbeing and quality of life. Ask yourself, 'Do my actions provide the support for my loved one to feel socially confident and that they are not alone?'

If you can, write this down or print it off; maybe put it on the fridge or somewhere else visible as a prompt to keep you on track. Everyone who interacts with your loved one can have a beneficial or negative effect, influencing how they feel and cope. Sharing the VIPS questions with wider family and friends will help to start conversations about how you all want to care and make the world a better place for everyone living with dementia.

In addition to supporting your loved one in line with the principles of person-centred care, the next most important principle of our approach is focusing on what is within your control.

FOCUS ON WHAT IS WITHIN YOUR CONTROL

Having a loved one receive a diagnosis of dementia can affect you in multiple ways: emotionally, psychologically, economically, socially, and physically. Many challenges can arise as your life and plans are interrupted by the implications of dementia and seeing its impact on your loved one. Life can really feel out of control and feeling anxious, angry, sad, frustrated, and overwhelmed are totally natural responses, not least given the stigma and misunderstandings that surround dementia.

It can be all too easy to get caught up in excessively worrying about things that are outside of your control: how quickly the dementia will progress, what the future will bring, how you will cope, and other worries. When things do not go the way you had planned or wanted, it can be all too easy to focus on things that you have no power over. You may then start ruminating about the things that aren't working in your favour, worrying about all the bad things that could happen next. This can cloud your judgement and leads to you losing a sense of your role in shaping your reality. Whilst it is completely natural to get lost in such worries, it is not useful or helpful. The more you focus on what is not within your control, the worse you will feel. So, the most important advice when supporting your loved one (or indeed for life in general) is to focus on what is within your control.

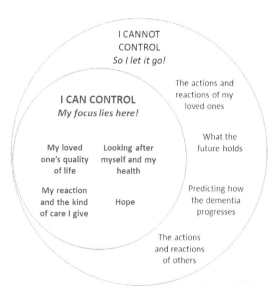

"*Happiness and freedom begin with a clear understanding of one principle: some things are within our control, and some things are not. The chief task in life is simply this: to identify and separate matters so that I can say clearly to myself, which are externals not under my control, and which have to do with the choices I actually control.*"

Epictetus (AD 50-135), philosopher[5]

Even when you feel you do not have any control in life, you have control over where you put your energies.

EXERCISE
Control in Your Life

Reflect on where you put your focus. Ask yourself these questions:

- Do you give your energy to factors that you cannot control?
- Do you wish or pray that your loved one did not have dementia?
- Do you conserve and direct your energy on to the areas that you are more likely to have some control over e.g., staying socially and physically active, eating well, stress management, making sure financial affairs are in order?

We will revisit this idea throughout the book, offering ideas about where you can focus your energies. You cannot control the future or get rid of your natural worries and feelings, just as you cannot control the progressive nature of dementia. However, you *can* control what you do, and there is a lot that can be done right now to improve your loved one's wellbeing as well as your own. Everything that follows offers you the opportunity to focus on things that you can control to better support your loved one's quality of life, whilst also managing your own health and wellbeing.

DEFINING YOUR SUPPORTING ROLE: THE POWER OF CHOICE

Before you read any further, take a few moments to digest what has been outlined so far. Do you want to explore and learn more about these ideas? Do they resonate with the kind of carer you would like to be? We appreciate that our approach may feel like a huge shift in understanding dementia. You may be feeling unsure, hopeful, or sceptical. When you feel ready to continue, it is now time to define your supporting role.

Let us return to the principle of focusing your energies where you do have some control. How you choose to frame dementia within the context of your life and that of your loved one is an important part of how you will manage this experience. Even though in your mind, other people and society may insist that dementia is a 'living death', you can choose to understand it differently, according to the principles of person-centred care (see page 7). Supporting your loved one will be less distressing if you choose to see dementia as a life-limiting condition as opposed to a 'loss of self' or a 'war'. There will be an infinite number of stories that can and will be told about dementia. Your story and that of your loved one are unique. By learning to think and speak about dementia differently, we can better support individuals and families coping with dementia. Whilst dementia will affect your loved one's abilities and self-awareness, this does not equate with their identity being destroyed or lost.

It is also completely natural to feel worried and overwhelmed when dementia comes into your life. However, you have a choice when it comes to your reactions. Do you choose to support and respond to your loved one with respect for their humanity, or with rejection and avoidance? If your decision is to try to support your loved one with respect and dignity, then we can offer plenty of strategies to help you along the way. By working with what dementia brings instead of fighting against it, and through focusing on your loved one's wellbeing and strengths, you can enable them to function at their best. Whilst caring for your loved one will invariably involve struggles at various points along the way, the experience can still be defined by deep emotional connections and meaningful opportunities.

BILL AND DOROTHY'S STORY

When Bill's wife Dorothy was first diagnosed with dementia, he felt worried and overwhelmed. They had no children and no other family living close by to help them. Bill decided he had a choice to make. He could let his worries get the better of him or he could choose to put his energies into doing what he could to support Dorothy as her needs increased. After all, this would be in the spirit of love and kindness and honouring the deep bond they had through 55 years of marriage. Although he felt exhausted at times, and the couple experienced many challenges, their lives were defined by emotional connection and a sense of purpose. Bill continued to attend the carer's group, which he said always helped to lift his spirits, whilst their neighbour spent time with Dorothy, which she enjoyed. Bill's choice to live in the spirit of love meant that dementia was only a chapter, rather than the whole story, in their long life together.

SUMMARY

With the challenges of caring for your loved one comes opportunities for personal growth. Your loved one can still offer you many opportunities to learn about yourself; as you adapt to changing demands, you will realize that you can do more than you first thought possible. Although implementing these ideas will require effort and adaptation, drawing on the principles of person-centred care will offer the best chance for your loved one to live a rich and dignified life at every stage of dementia, and for you to derive a sense of purpose and meaning alongside them.

KEY POINTS TO REMEMBER

- There will be an infinite number of stories that can be told about dementia. Your story and that of your loved one are unique.
- Person-centred care offers you opportunities to focus your efforts and improve your loved one's wellbeing and bring meaning to the caring role with dignity and respect.
- Focus on what is within your control.
- Whilst caring for your loved one will involve challenges, the experience can still be defined by deep emotional connections.

"We cannot change the cards we are dealt, just how we play the hand."

Randy Pausch, *The Last Lecture*[6]

CHAPTER 2

WHAT IS DEMENTIA?

"We lament the millions of neurons lost to dementia and ignore the many millions that work perfectly well."

Dr Allen Power, geriatrician and board member of
US Dementia Action Alliance

Do you ever wonder why your loved one can tell you in detail about some distant event, but cannot remember what they had for breakfast? Or perhaps you wonder about how dementia changes over time and what to expect. This chapter will give an overview of dementia more generally. Although each person's condition progresses differently, having a better understanding of dementia will help you to prepare, adjust your expectations and support your loved one's changing needs over time.

True or False?
Dementia is more than memory loss.

This statement is true. Dementia is a syndrome – usually of a chronic or progressive nature – in which there is deterioration in cognitive function (i.e., the brain-based skills and abilities) beyond what might be expected from normal ageing. As well as memory loss, thinking; understanding; language; concentration; and judgement can all be affected. Changes in motivation and emotional responses may also arise and a person may have less control over their feelings and how they express them.

There are many different forms of dementia. Alzheimer's disease is the most common and perhaps most well-known type; others can be broadly labelled as vascular dementia, dementia with Lewy bodies, Parkinson's disease dementia, and frontotemporal dementias. The boundaries between different subtypes of dementia are indistinct and mixed forms often co-exist. Dementia is one of the major causes of disability and dependency among older people worldwide. As dementia progresses, increasing levels of care will be required.

HOW COMMON IS DEMENTIA?

Although you may feel very alone at times, many people all over the world are also living with or supporting a loved one with dementia. The World Health Organization (WHO) estimates that over 50 million people worldwide are living with dementia, with nearly 10 million new cases every year. The estimated proportion of the general population aged 60 and over with dementia at a given time is between 5–8 per cent. More women are affected by dementia than men; worldwide, women with dementia outnumber men 2 to 1.

HOW DO YOU GET DEMENTIA?

True or False?
Dementia is a normal part of ageing.

This statement is false. Although age is the strongest known risk factor, dementia is not an inevitable consequence of getting older and does not only affect older people. Young-onset dementia (before the age of 65) accounts for up to 9 per cent of people with dementia. When it comes to why more women develop dementia, the role of hormonal factors amongst other variables affecting brain health and brain ageing appear to play a central role.[7,8] Everyone's brain ages along a different trajectory. Some brains age along a gentle curve, others curve slowly and dip at the end, whilst other brains age more rapidly and earlier.[9]

Genetics and environmental factors play a part along with lifestyle and medical factors. Studies estimate that at least one-third of dementia cases could be prevented by attending to lifestyle and medical factors.[10] The risk of dementia can be reduced by eating a healthy diet, controlling weight, getting regular exercise, reducing alcohol intake, and not smoking. It is important to balance hormones and maintain healthy blood pressure, cholesterol, and blood-sugar levels, which can compromise blood circulation to the brain. Depression, chronic stress, and social isolation are also risk factors for developing dementia and therefore social engagement and stress reduction play a protective role. We will discuss physical health issues further in Chapters 4 and 5 and how they relate to you and your loved one.

WHAT ARE THE SYMPTOMS OF DEMENTIA?

Dementia affects each person in different ways, depending on the type(s) of dementia, the person's personality before developing the disease, other health conditions, lifestyle, social supports, and their environment. A person's insight into their difficulties can also vary; your loved one may notice their difficulties, or they may not. It may be that you are more aware of the changes than they are. The table below outlines some of these changes.

Changes in Thinking and Memory	Changes in Behaviour and Mood	Changes in Daily Living Tasks and Physical Health
Memory	Personality	Self-care
Disorientation	Depression	Mobility, movement, balance and coordination
Confusion	Anxiety	Continence
New learning	Apathy	Financial management
Word finding	Frustration and anger	Health and medications
Language	Sleep disturbance	Food, diet, eating and swallowing
Thinking speed	Hallucinations	Household management
Understanding	Delusions	Driving and travel
Reasoning and judgement	Social skills and abilities	
Visuospatial abilities (judging depth, and distance perception)		

Your loved one may not experience all these changes and the degree to which they are experienced will differ between individuals.

DEMENTIA'S JOURNEY

We will be focusing on the changes associated with dementia in more detail in later chapters. Before we move on, it can help to understand the progression of dementia in three broad stages: from early to middle to late stages. Just as dementia affects each person in different ways, these stages can also vary in length and intensity. Some types of dementia progress slowly, whilst others progress more rapidly. Again, due to the unique nature of each person's circumstances there is no way of knowing or predicting the rate of dementia progression.

Early Stages: The early stages of dementia can be overlooked, and the signs dismissed as 'senior moments' when the onset is very gradual and subtle. Common symptoms include:

- Forgetfulness e.g., of recent events
- Difficulty learning new information
- Losing track of the time
- Trouble concentrating
- Anxiety and low mood

Middle Stages: As dementia progresses to the middle stages, the signs and symptoms become more noticeable, compromising a person's ability to maintain their previous levels of independence. Symptoms can include:

- Becoming more forgetful of recent events and people's names
- Misplacing things at home or getting lost in familiar places
- Previously simple tasks, such as cooking a meal or going to buy groceries, may become more difficult due to memory and organizational difficulties.

- Problems managing finances
- Problems travelling to new locations without getting lost
- Increasing difficulty with communication, such as finding the right word
- Withdrawing from social interactions because of communication and memory problems
- Living as if in the past; believing home is where they lived 20 years ago, difficulty remembering that significant others have died e.g., their parents
- Needing increased levels of support with personal care and daily activities
- Behaviour and mood changes
- Movement difficulties – coordination and balance may be compromised (although in some types of dementia these difficulties can appear in the earlier stages)

Later Stages: As dementia progresses to the later stages, cognitive disturbances are serious, and the physical signs and symptoms become more obvious. Greatly reduced activity levels and dependence on others for most, if not all, personal care will be required. Symptoms can include:

- Becoming unaware of time and place
- Communication may be primarily through behaviours, gestures, and feelings
- Having difficulty recognizing relatives and friends

- Higher dependence on others for care and daily activities
- Movement difficulties and increased frailty
- Behaviour and mood changes

HOW IS DEMENTIA TREATED?

True or False?
There is nothing that can be done to improve a person with
dementia's quality of life.

This statement is false. Although there are medications to help with some of the symptoms of dementia, there are no medical treatments currently available to cure the diseases underlying the most common types of dementia or to alter the progressive course. However, by adopting a person-centred approach that focuses on the uniqueness of each individual and improving lifestyle factors, you can significantly improve your loved one's quality of life, health, mood and wellbeing, which will be discussed in the chapters that follow. The field of medicine is also moving toward a more personalized and person-centred approach, recognizing the importance of this. Precision medicine focuses on the uniqueness of each individual, looking at their particular genetics, lifestyle and environment and allowing for far more effective strategies for disease prevention and treatment rather than the traditional 'one-size fits all' approach.

A CHANGE OF FOCUS

Changing your approach can improve your loved one's wellbeing better than any medications or other treatments. Learning to focus on the things that matter to you and your loved one, alongside interests and strengths, will help to improve quality of life for you both. We explore how to do this in more detail throughout the book.

As outlined in Chapter 1, the way your loved one feels, and how they experience life, is down to much more than just having dementia. There are many factors that play a significant role in wellbeing, with personal relationships and social environment being central. Many people with dementia see their life as far from over; rather there is an increased focus on the 'here-and-now', and a particular wisdom from dealing more directly with grief and loss. Despite the changes arising from dementia, your loved one will still feel an emotional connection to people and their environment, even in the later stages. With support and understanding, they can adapt to changing perceptions.

- Focus on what your loved one *can do*, rather than on what they can no longer do.
- Focus on how they *feel*, rather than what they remember (or cannot remember).

This different focus will help you both to live better with dementia.

"Changing your approach can improve your loved one's wellbeing better than any medications or other treatments."

EXERCISE
A Different Focus

Take a journal or a piece of paper and list some of your loved one's strengths, qualities, and abilities. Do this with your loved one if they are able to, and want to join in. Think broadly e.g., sense of humour to kindness, a sense of adventure or love of family to skills, anything from giving great hugs or making things.

SUMMARY

Dementia comprises a range of diseases that affect brain functioning. For most people, the risk of developing dementia is due to a combination of unique genetic makeup, medical health, the environment, and lifestyle. Dementia affects each person in different ways. This will depend on the type(s) of dementia, the person's personality before developing the disease and other health conditions, lifestyle, social supports, and their environment. As dementia progresses, your loved one will require increasing levels of care. Having a better understanding of dementia will help you to prepare, adjust your expectations, and support your loved one's changing needs over time. Adopting a person-centred approach will offer significant benefits for your loved one's mood and wellbeing over time.

KEY POINTS TO REMEMBER

- Many people with dementia see their life as far from over.
- Despite the changes arising from dementia, your loved one will still feel an emotional connection to people and their environment, even in the later stages.
- Changing your approach and making lifestyle changes can improve your loved one's wellbeing better than any medications or other treatments offered.
- Learning to focus on the things that matter to you and your loved one, alongside their interests and strengths, will help to improve quality of life for you both.

CHAPTER 3

YOUR ROLE

"Do the best you can until you know better. Then when you know better, do better."

Maya Angelou, American poet and civil rights activist

Have you ever found yourself arguing with your loved one over their difficulties; you trying to convince them of their diagnosis, them having none of it? Or maybe you have found yourself trying to convince other family members of your loved one's diagnosis, only to be told, 'Don't be silly, Mum is fine.' Do these experiences sound familiar? If so, then this chapter may resonate. Accepting a diagnosis of dementia can be challenging – for everyone. Denial is a common experience. Coming to terms with the diagnosis and learning to accept the changes and limitations that your loved one experiences over time is a critical factor in managing the caring role. In this chapter, we will also explore values in relation to this role – who and what do you want to stand for as a carer? Clarifying your values can help to keep you on track when supporting your loved one, in line with the principles of person-centred care, as outlined in Chapter 1.

COMING TO TERMS WITH THE DIAGNOSIS

Everyone's experience of getting a dementia diagnosis will differ; some people may feel relieved, others may be in shock, others may refuse to believe the diagnosis. Denial can result in an inability or unwillingness to talk about your loved one's difficulties, perhaps believing the diagnosis is wrong.

It is understandable that getting a dementia diagnosis, or that of any life-limiting or terminal condition, can result in shock and denial. It may feel that your hopes and dreams for the future are dashed. A dementia diagnosis is not on anyone's list of hopes, and it can take time to come to terms with – people will adjust at their own pace. Dementia can be considered an 'invisible illness' because it is not outwardly visible, and this can make it harder to accept. Nevertheless, learning to accept the diagnosis is important. It will help you to better understand the changes your loved one is going through and manage your expectations, which can greatly reduce frustration and stress, as well as help you to start adjusting to the caring role and support your loved one as they get their affairs in order.

YOUR LOVED ONE'S ACCEPTANCE OF THE DIAGNOSIS

Being diagnosed with dementia can be frightening and devastating, particularly in the early days when the person may still be able to comprehend things well and therefore have a greater understanding of the disease and its implications. There are several reasons why it may be difficult for your loved one to accept their diagnosis:

- Their fear acts as a psychological coping mechanism. If they don't accept that there is a problem, then the reality can be avoided – 'If I ignore it, it will go away.' Ignorance is bliss.
- Many people go through a sort of grieving process, and a part of it is denial. Anger, resentment, guilt, and sadness are also all normal responses.
- As dementia progresses, the part of the brain that understands there is a problem becomes compromised, and so your loved one may not be able to fully comprehend or recognize their difficulties.
- Their ability to remember their difficulties will also become compromised. They may know and feel something is wrong, but have difficulty processing this due to cognitive changes.

All these factors can be hard for you as a carer when you can see so clearly the changes in your loved one's abilities. However, you cannot force or persuade them to accept their symptoms. In this instance, the single most effective coping strategy is for you to accept your loved one's inability to recognize they have dementia. This saves countless struggles and indeed arguments, trying to persuade and convince them. It is not the same as hiding the diagnosis from your loved one. It is essential that they are part of the assessment and diagnostic process.

"Your loved one does not have to accept that they have dementia for you to find ways to help them."

The good news is that they do not have to accept that they have dementia for you to find ways to help them. Therefore, it is simply not necessary to remind your loved one repeatedly of their diagnosis. Realizing this can help you to feel more compassion and less frustration with their difficulties and changing abilities.

DAVID'S STORY

David's children asked, 'How can we help Dad to understand and accept that he has dementia? He keeps saying nothing is wrong with him even though the doctor told him he has dementia, and he blames everyone else for moving his glasses and taking his money when he misplaces them.' This was leading to an unhelpful power struggle, where everyone was frustrated. Through dementia education, David's children learned that they did not need their father to accept his diagnosis to support him, and rather than get into arguments about them not taking his glasses or wallet, they would simply help him to find them without making a big deal about it.

YOUR ABILITY TO ACCEPT THE DIAGNOSIS

As you are reading this book, the chances are you have already accepted that your loved one has dementia. However, this acceptance can be an ongoing process, and at times, it will feel like a struggle. You may worry that it means you are giving up on your loved one. Given the common negative stereotypes of dementia, outlined in Chapter 1, acceptance of it can feel terrifying – it is human nature to deny and avoid what we find frightening. However, when fear prevents us from facing reality, it does not help anyone. Believing your loved one will get better can result in them being denied the support they need. Drawing on the ideas outlined, it is better if you can, to believe that your loved one can *live well* with dementia.

Accepting a diagnosis when your loved one is in the earlier stages of dementia can be particularly challenging. The change in their abilities may be quite gradual, as outlined in Chapter 2, and subtle to the point that you may sometimes doubt there are any difficulties at all. There may be inconsistency, with good days followed by not so good days.

It usually follows that with acceptance of dementia comes greater acceptance of your loved one's limitations and decreasing control over their actions, which helps to reduce frustration and blame. Being able to take a step back and see their struggles as part of the changes in their brain can help you to take things less personally and to have more realistic expectations of them.

> "It usually follows that with acceptance of dementia comes greater acceptance of your loved one's limitations."

Practical Considerations

By accepting the diagnosis, you can seek the right help and support and begin to plan ahead. It is important to put legal, health, and financial plans in place whilst your loved one can still participate in the process. You may need to consider home adaptations and safety measures to reduce risks, look at medical choices, and make decisions regarding property and finances. Although we cannot control the future, supporting your loved one as they get their affairs in order will go some way to ensuring their wishes are respected and brings everyone some peace of mind. Many documents can be prepared without the help of legal services. However, if you are unsure about how to complete legal documents or make financial plans, you may want to seek assistance from a solicitor or financial advisor who is familiar with dementia and advanced care planning. See page 215 for an Advance Directive template, which outlines your loved one's wishes for future health and medical decisions.

If your loved one drives, this will also need to be considered in terms of safety. Please seek advice regarding driving and dementia from the relevant agencies, and your loved one's doctor, as guidelines may vary from country to country.

GOPAL'S STORY

Following his diagnosis of dementia, Gopal and his family began to discuss planning for the future, notably his wishes regarding his finances and health. Gopal was clear that he wanted his wife and son to act on his behalf if he could no longer make decisions for himself, both with regards to his finances and decisions regarding his health. Although it was difficult to have these conversations as a family, everyone felt some relief afterwards, knowing that they could respect Gopal's wishes when required.

Alongside planning ahead, accepting your loved one has dementia can also help to prioritize their wishes for the present – what do they want to do now, while they are able?

WHEN FAMILY AND FRIENDS STRUGGLE TO ACCEPT DEMENTIA

It may be that each member of the family has a different opinion and perspective about what has changed, or has not, and what should be done. As with grief and loss, everyone will have a unique response to the acceptance of the diagnosis. It can be very painful seeing a loved one struggle and some family members and friends may withdraw to protect their feelings. This can result in the loss of opportunities to create special memories, leading to potential guilt and regret later.

"As with grief and loss, everyone will have a unique response to the acceptance of the diagnosis."

Conflict in the Family

Denial on the part of a family member can be a major source of stress and frustration for those who are left facing the reality, and this can lead to conflict. The person in denial may not help while you, having accepted the diagnosis, take on multiple demands, sometimes alone. You may be accused of 'overreacting' when trying to explain the difficulties faced by your loved one and the support they need. Family members in denial may obstruct extra care and insist that your loved one can still live independently. This can be frustrating and risky, leaving you feeling unsupported and isolated. You may find it helpful to provide family members with reading materials about dementia or direct them to online resources that they can look at and process in their own time (see Appendices). Having these conversations with professionals present may also help it to feel less confrontational.

HOW TO HELP

Here are some tips to help others accept the diagnosis:

- Try to be gentle and calm. Anger will only result in conflict.
- Explain that it is understandable that they are frightened or worried – perhaps share some of your own feelings and your fears, as well as hopes.
- Let your family member or friend know that they are not alone.
- Explain that denial and doing nothing will result in more problems for everyone, rather than helping anyone.
- If they do not accept it, let it go – you can always return to it another time.
- It can be challenging if a family member has had a difficult relationship with your loved one, so hold this in mind when managing expectations.

BECOMING INFORMED

There are many dementia organizations with local branches worldwide that provide information and peer support to help people come to terms with the diagnosis and access help. Finding out what local community resources are available can be a big help when it comes to managing anxiety and worries about the future. If local support is not available, national and international organizations can also offer a lot of advice and signposting, in addition to connecting you with other carers. Make a note of helpful resources. You will find a range of these organizations listed in Useful Resources.

YOUR VALUES

As you come to terms with your loved one having dementia and, consequently, their increased reliance on you, the next step is to focus on what kind of carer you want to be. Identifying and clarifying the values that influence your decisions and behaviour will help you to adjust to your loved one's changing needs and support them in a way that is consistent with the person you want to be in life. Being clear about what you want to stand for as a carer will help you to feel a sense of purpose and continue to support your loved one, despite the sadness and worry you may feel at times. Without a sense of purpose, it can be all too easy to give up and feel defeated when things do not go according to plan. Some days you may feel that you cannot do right for doing wrong. On these occasions, you can go back to your values and the principles of person-centred care and find a sense of purpose, even in the face of pain and challenges.

EXERCISE
Meaning and Purpose

Answer these questions to consider what brings meaning and purpose in your life:

- What gives you a sense of purpose?
- What do you stand for?
- Do you have a specific aim that is important to you?
- Has the diagnosis of dementia affected your attitude to the future?
- What worries you the most about the future?

SO, WHAT ARE VALUES?

- Values can be understood as your heart's deepest desire for how you want to behave as a human being.
  What kind of person do you want to be as you support your loved one?
- Values are not about what you want to get or achieve; they are about how you want to act on an ongoing basis; how

you want to treat yourself, others, and the world around you. In effect, values are like a compass that guides you in the direction you want to go.[11]

- Values may feel instinctual, they can be cultural, and sometimes they become apparent by chance or through experiences.

- Values are also flexible. The context determines which values you will act upon in any given moment. For example, you may choose to act with assertiveness regarding your loved one's treatment and care. Going back to the principle of focusing your energies where you have more control, you have more control over your actions than your thoughts and feelings. For example, whilst you may feel angry when your loved one has asked you the same question repeatedly, you can still choose to act with kindness and understanding toward them (whilst taking a deep breath).

- It is also important to differentiate values from goals. Values are about *how* you want to behave (e.g., with patience), and goals are about what you want to get or achieve (e.g., optimizing your loved one's quality of life).

THE THREE Cs

There are many examples of values – being assertive, adventurous, kind, forgiving, curious, and so on. Some will resonate, others will not. Whilst many words can describe values,

Dr Russ Harris, an Australian-based medical practitioner and ACT psychotherapist, helpfully groups values into three main headings: Connection, Caring and Contribution – the three Cs.[12] These words can be a helpful starting point when considering your values.

The three Cs are core to the principles of person-centred care, and so they can offer reassurance that you are on the right track when supporting your loved one. These values can also help to guide how you look after yourself, which we will explore in Chapter 5. We will look at each of these in turn, linking them back to the VIPS model (see page 12).

Connection – Being in the Moment

Connection can be defined as being fully present, right here and now, and engaged psychologically and emotionally with your loved one. Being connected and attuned to them will help you to understand their changing needs. This becomes even more important when language abilities deteriorate. Being connected is the opposite of being distracted, which compromises the care and understanding that can be provided. Instead of worrying about the future or dwelling on the past, you are focused and engaged with the present moment. Returning to the VIPS model, the value of connection can be reframed as:

- 'Do I make a serious attempt to see my actions from my loved one's perspective or standpoint?'
- 'Do I recognize my loved one's individual uniqueness?'

"Being connected and attuned becomes even more important when your loved one's language abilities deteriorate."

Caring – Bringing Warmth

Relationships will not thrive or survive in the absence of care. When we genuinely care and act in ways that show kindness and compassion, our relationships will feel secure. In contrast, when we act in ways that are neglectful and uncaring, our relationships will suffer. Reframing the value of caring within the VIPS model:

- 'Do my actions value and honour my loved one as they live with dementia?'

Contribution – Offering a Hand

Relationships thrive when we contribute to them by offering support, care, and help. Investing in our relationships helps them to flourish. Finally, reframing contribution within the VIPS model:

- 'Do my actions provide the support for my loved one to feel socially confident and that they are not alone?'

EXERCISE
Values and Caring

- What can you do, at this very moment, in this relationship, that involves caring, connection and contribution?
- Can you be open to your loved one's feelings, thoughts and needs?
- What can you do to show that you care?
- What can you do to contribute to their wellbeing at this moment in time?

Try to slow down, be open and curious, pay more attention to your loved one's face, eyes, tone of voice, posture, and what they are saying in trying to communicate.

COMMITTED ACTION

Once you feel that you have a clear sense of the values that you wish to live by, the next step is to translate them into committed action. While clarifying your values is essential, it will mean very little at the end of the day if there is no action taken to live by those values. A rich and meaningful life is developed by taking effective action that is guided and motivated by your values.[13]

Next, we will look at the keys areas that you can focus your energies on, drawing on these values to take action and achieve the goal of improving your loved one's quality of life.

SUMMARY

Everyone's experience of getting a dementia diagnosis will differ and processing this can take time. Denial is a common response. Learning to accept that your loved one has dementia is a key step for making future plans and prioritizing current life wishes, as well as managing the expectations of your loved one and yourself. This will help to reduce risks and enable you to seek appropriate help and support. Accepting the changing nature of your loved one's limitations as their dementia progresses can be difficult; no sooner do you feel you have adjusted, then things can change again. Although it can be disconcerting and painful as you adjust, drawing on your values will help you to find purpose in this journey, even in the face of challenges, and take action to improve your loved one's wellbeing.

KEY POINTS TO REMEMBER

- Acceptance of dementia benefits everyone, helping to manage expectations, plan for the future, and adjust to the changes it brings over time.
- If your loved one does not appear to accept that they have dementia, do not become preoccupied with this.

- Clarify your values and use these to guide how you support your loved one and optimize their quality of life.
- No matter how many times you feel you fall short, you can reassess your actions according to your values and set realistic goals regarding your loved one's care and wellbeing.

CHAPTER 4

QUALITY OF LIFE AND WELLBEING

"There is a reason I am drawn to this field. It's because people living with dementia have a lot to teach me."

Dr Elaine Eshbaugh, US-based Professor of
Gerontology and Family Studies

Maintaining a good quality of life is possible following a diagnosis of dementia. In this chapter, we will help you to support your loved one's wellbeing, drawing on your values and the principles of person-centred care, as outlined in Chapters 1 and 3. Despite the changes that dementia brings, your loved one can continue to lead a productive, satisfying life. It is important that they are helped to feel they can still make a difference and contribute to family and friends' lives.

Some people think that once a person is diagnosed with dementia, they are no longer capable of doing the normal activities they once did, but in the earlier stages, they can. In fact, although adjustments and assistance will be required as dementia progresses, your loved one can continue to engage in meaningful activities and maintain a sense of connection, caring and contribution right until the end of their life. Supporting your loved one's wellbeing may come easily, or it may take some discovery together to find new areas of life that can bring fulfillment. This chapter will give you some ideas so that you can focus your energy on where you have more control, and improve your loved one's wellbeing.

ASSESSING QUALITY OF LIFE

It is understandable that you may view your loved one's quality of life from your own worried, stressed perspective and make assumptions about it, but that can vary significantly from how they see it and experience it themselves. Quality of life is defined by each individual and their unique circumstances, not their dementia. Therefore, rather than making assumptions, it is important to take the time to ask your loved one for their views and what matters to them. Remember Social GRRAACCEESS (see page 10) and the many aspects of difference within our personal and social identities? There are many factors outside a person's dementia that affect their quality of life, which can be improved and changed. The type of care your loved one receives, as well as their living environment, will greatly influence their sense of identity, and the purpose and pleasure they can continue to get from life.

Flexibility as circumstances inevitably shift and change is also important. Although everyone may define 'quality of life' somewhat differently depending on individual preferences, likes and dislikes, there are some common factors that are true for most people. The following section elaborates on the factors that have been identified by people with dementia as being important to their wellbeing and quality of life. These factors include relationships, identity, meaningful activities, and health. Expectations regarding what is possible within each of these factors can be adjusted according to your loved one's changing needs, interests and abilities.

RELATIONSHIPS

Relationships naturally change through life and living with dementia means adapting to yet more change. Having someone to talk to, and maintaining relationships, is rated as the most important factor in facilitating quality of life for people with dementia. People who are living with dementia have an unchanged basic human need to have relationships with others. However, maintaining relationships can become difficult due to the changes associated with dementia. It is important to attend to different aspects of relationships, including sexual needs and intimacy. For partners, the expression of affection for each other may change, but it is possible to discover new and different ways of being intimate and sharing closeness. It can be useful to have a broad definition of intimacy and sex, and permissions and consent checking may also require more attention. You know your loved one best and so you will know the signs if discomfort or pleasure arise.

With planning and support, your loved one can maintain positive relationships with family, friends, and wider social networks, and this will help to reduce the risk of isolation, depression, and social withdrawal.

When there is a lot to be done, it can be easy to overlook the need to just sit down and talk with each other. Make a conscious effort to slow down and take an unhurried approach to time spent together. Give your loved one the time they need and try to focus on the present moment. Although it can be difficult to see the brighter side of life at times, humour is valued by people with dementia. Share a joke or laugh at yourself. Laughter is clinically proven to be good medicine, so have fun where possible.

"It was magical to be able to open her Mother's Day pressies, have a giggle over silly things and engage in idle 'chit chat'. We love silly jokes too. I played music on my phone and it was great when mum started to sing along to a few of her favourite tunes."
Shirley

INTERACTING WITH CHILDREN

Children can play a big role in dementia care. Discovering opportunities for your loved one and children to connect meaningfully through person-centred activities that are engaging for both ages can have mutual benefits. Many people living with dementia experience high levels of positive engagement and a sense of worth when interacting with children. Both can appreciate living in the moment, which brings a whole new relationship and experience. Children do not have the prejudices and fears that adults have, and they can be more accepting; they can also develop new life experiences because of these interactions, which are a fundamental part of their learning and development.

"Children do not have the prejudices and fears that adults do, and they can be more accepting."

THE BENEFITS OF PETS

Pets can be invaluable for improving quality of life for people with dementia. Benefits include:

- Companionship
- Improved mood and health
- Opportunities for physical activity
- A sense of purpose from caring for them, all without the need for language
- As dementia progresses, the physical touch of stroking a pet can continue to bring an enormous sense of wellbeing and calm.

IDENTITY AND LIFE STORY

Dr Richard Taylor, an American clinical psychologist, founded the Dementia Alliance International (DAI) after being diagnosed with dementia aged 58. He began writing about his fears and triumphs to "gain control over what was happening between my ears" and "to reassure myself that some of the old me was still there, because I was in transition in ways no one seemed to understand". He advocated for the recognition of people with dementia "as whole and complete human beings who also happen to be living with a chronic disability". Finding ways to support and preserve your loved one's identity is an important part of the caring role. Whilst reminiscing and reflecting on the past can facilitate a better understanding of your loved one's life before dementia, it will become increasingly important as the dementia progresses to help maintain and sustain your loved one's sense of self and identity in the present. "We need support to stay in today," Dr Taylor urges. "Staying in the past is not the highest priority for any human being."[14]

Everyone is engaged in an ongoing process of constructing a life story, or personal narrative, that determines their self-understanding and position in the world. This is no different when a person develops dementia. It is the words we use, and the stories we tell about ourselves and others, that create our psychological and social realities (see Chapter 1). Narrative approaches offer a powerful means to support your loved one's identity and identify what is important to enable preferred ways of living,[15] despite the progressive nature of dementia.

TREE OF LIFE

Developing a Tree of Life book is a collaborative process with your loved one, family and friends. You can use images, photos, music, anything that helps to bring their life story to life, which can be revisited over time.

This is a narrative approach developed by Ncazelo Ncube and David Denborough, African and Australian-based therapists. Ncube says that the Tree of Life is an opportunity to create a second story about your life and to make sure people have a "safe place to stand in relation to the problems and challenges they face …".[16] We often use this approach to support identity and wellbeing of the people we work with.

> *"The Tree of Life is a brilliant experience. It brings awareness to the type of person you are – the whole of me. I had forgotten about all the positives about myself. After the experience and revisiting the tree, I feel honest and proud of what I do."*
> *Patrisha*

Supporting your loved one to share their stories can enhance their sense of identity and connection to you and others, and to their wider life beyond dementia. The following ideas are drawn from the Tree of Life approach and are a helpful place to start with your loved one, but there are no limits. You can compile the following online, or in a book or journal, so that it can be shared with permission:

- The here and now. Where your loved one lives, the daily activities and interests they enjoy.
- Consider your loved one's past. Discuss childhood and middle years; their heritage, family, culture, country/place of origin, events and places of significance, religion, values, traditions, favourite childhood songs and games, important people.

- Explore strengths, skills, talents, important characteristics, and abilities. If you find this difficult, think about what other people have said about your loved one. What qualities and skills are admired? (e.g., being kind and caring). Pick up on skills you may have observed, and discuss specific examples.
- Your loved one's hopes, dreams and wishes, however big or small.
- Significant people, pets, and animals, past and present, real or fictional.
- Gifts they have been given, both material and non-material. Examples include love, care, support, creativity, their grandmother's ring, their father's watch.
- Gifts they have given others, both material and non-material. This might include the gift of life, fun and laughter, delicious cakes, cosy knits.
- Difficult times that lie ahead alongside generating solutions and problem-solving together. This helps to bring a sense of agency and collaboration.

"Supporting your loved one to share their stories can enhance their sense of identity and connection to you and others."

Due to changes in your loved one's memory and language abilities, they may need help to communicate important aspects of their identity. This is the beauty of a Tree of Life as it documents what is important to the person and what they want others to know about them.

As your loved one's needs and preferences may change over time, do update any written documents pertaining to these and share with relevant others as required. This will help to support person-centred care as dementia progresses and verbal communication deteriorates. This will also be helpful if your loved one requires formal carers in the home or subsequently moves into a residential or care facility (see Chapter 8).

MEANINGFUL ACTIVITIES AND ENJOYING THE MOMENT

Everyone wants to feel useful, and this is no different when a person develops dementia. We have previously discussed the importance of developing an understanding of what is important to your loved one, within their life context. Support activities that fit their likes, and avoid their dislikes. Keep in mind that just because your loved one did an activity in their past, it does not mean they enjoyed it. They may have done it out of obligation, so ask them and gauge their interest. Activities become much more meaningful when they are things the person has previously enjoyed – and activities that bear little relevance to your loved one's interests may result in distress and irritation.

HOW TO HELP

Below are some ideas that may offer more meaningful engagement for your loved one. When looking at each activity, consider your loved one's stage of dementia, preferences and interests, and ensure they are safe and comfortable. Remember, activities may only last for a few minutes; they don't have to be complicated. Ideally, have a selection of activities to hand.

Household tasks: Baking, cooking, laundry, gardening, cleaning, polishing, knitting, sewing, weaving.

Games and puzzles: Jigsaws, board games, cards, word puzzles.

Arts and crafts: Painting, colouring, papercrafts, pottery.

Reminiscence: Photo albums, life story books, memory box containing memorabilia of hobbies, objects of interest e.g., coin collection, postcards from holidays.

Apps: Brain training, relaxation, games, reminiscence.

Sensory stimulation: Sensory rooms and gardens, music, audiobooks, virtual museum tours, movies and musicals, hand massage, spa days, rummage bag (a bag or box of interesting objects and textures), comfortable or weighted blankets.

Physical activity: Walks in the garden, walks indoors, chair-based exercise, housework, cleaning, dancing, Tai Chi, yoga.

Music: Radio, TV, records, tapes, CDs, apps, YouTube.

It is important to recognize that some activities that your loved one enjoyed earlier in life may now result in confusion or frustration. As dementia progresses, it may take some trial, error, and creativity to find interests, hobbies or pastimes that work well. Adapting them to meet your loved one's unique needs and abilities can be a process, but patience will be rewarded. When considering meaningful activities:

- Aim for a balance of stimulation and interest, so that your loved one can feel engaged without being over-or under-stimulated.
- Offer some choice.
- Choose activities that are not too simple or overly complicated. The best activities provide a challenge, while also giving a sense of accomplishment. Those that are too simple will inevitably result in boredom and under-stimulation. Activities that are too difficult may result in your loved one becoming frustrated and defeated.
- Keep alert to changing needs over time and day to day, depending on how tired your loved one may be.

WINSTON'S STORY

Winston had always loved reading and doing word searches and crosswords. His daughter Brenda noticed that he appeared to be losing interest in these activities a few years after developing dementia. She took him to the optician to check his glasses were correct and then bought books with bigger print and puzzles at increasingly easier levels, which they often did together. Brenda also got Winston audiobooks from the library, which he enjoyed listening to, right through to the advanced stages of dementia.

Although your loved one will require increasing levels of supervision and help, it is important to remember that they are an adult who has lived a long, purposeful life, and not to treat them like a child.

- There is no 'right' and 'wrong' with how activities are performed. It is the process of engagement that matters. Try to allow room for creativity.
- Engaging in meaningful activities is about self-expression in that moment, rather than being about the end-product or result. Try to guide your loved one when they need it, without assisting unless asked.

Taking over when it is not needed can result in feelings of helplessness and depression due to everything being done for them.

- Don't force your loved one to participate in activities they do not want to do. Resist the urge to give your loved one tasks just to occupy their time. Being engaged in meaningful activities is far more important than just keeping busy for the sake of it. This can feel like a delicate balance between supporting your loved one enough to maintain their interest and wellbeing, whilst allowing for quiet and rest if that is needed.

MUSIC AND ART

Music and art allow for self-expression and engagement, including in the advanced stages of dementia. Music is a powerful connector, which can bring people together in the here and now. The universal nature of the ability to enjoy music provides a powerful tool to enhance the quality of life of people with dementia, at little to no cost. Listening to music that spans your loved one's life can help to trigger memories, which can also help to stimulate conversations.

"'Happy Days are Here Again", "Oh I Do Like to Be Beside the Seaside" and "Quando, Quando, Quando" are my mum's favourites. Mum has a wonderful time singing away.

Of course, I join in too! I must admit hearing mum singing and seeing her do her 'shoulder shimmy' to the music in person, is the moment that reduces me to happy tears! WOW – it's unbeatable – music is the best. What a perfect day!'"
Shirley and her mother, Eileen

Music can support people living with dementia to communicate beyond words. It supports emotional health and wellbeing, particularly at a time when emotions can be overwhelming or difficult to process or manage. Studies have shown music can help to reduce agitation, low mood and anxiety. You can help your loved one to make a playlist of music they enjoy. Dancing and movement also offer multiple health benefits that do not rely on memory or language; rather they focus on strengths, feelings, and ongoing abilities, which can be adapted to chair-based movement as frailty increases. Painting and drawing can help with non-verbal communication when verbal communication is more difficult. There are also the sensory benefits of paint, paper craft and pottery. Use of art materials can stimulate the imagination and help your loved one to feel more connected to the world and people around them.

SPIRITUALITY

If spirituality and faith are important to a person, they do not go away with a diagnosis of dementia. If your loved one's faith is important to them, they might enjoy listening to prayers and sermons on the TV, radio, or internet. Hymns, chants and mantras that are performed with instruments may help with relaxation and provide a sense of calm.

HOW TO HELP

Using the points in this chapter, make a list in a notebook or your journal of some of the things your loved one enjoyed in the past, and new ideas if these have changed:

- What kind of things did your loved one enjoy before their diagnosis?
- Was there a certain type of music they appreciated?
- Did they enjoy sports, going for walks or dancing?
- Perhaps they enjoyed gazing out of the window at nature, loved the night sky or digging in the garden?
- Is your loved one a people person or do they prefer their own company?
- Which of these interests can you do together?
- What can they do with other people? What can they do alone?

PHYSICAL HEALTH

The key to living well with dementia is staying healthy – physically and mentally. It will be easier for your loved one to take on new challenges and lead a meaningful life when they feel well in themselves. A good diet, adequate hydration, exercise, sleeping well, and being free of pain and infection are critical in maintaining good health and wellbeing.

As dementia progresses, your loved one may become less able to identify health problems or to tell others about them, so it is important to look out for signs that they might be in pain or discomfort (see Chapter 7).

SLEEP AND DEMENTIA

Almost 50 per cent of people living with dementia experience sleep disturbance. This can include:

- Shorter sleep cycles with greater sleep disturbance.
- Less deep and REM (rapid eye movement) sleep, with reduced sleep efficiency.
- More frequent night-time waking, wandering and increased daytime napping.
- More difficulty falling asleep.
- 'Sundowning' occurs when the person becomes more restless, anxious, or agitated during the late afternoon and evening hours because their internal body clock is affected by the dementia process. This may take effect between the hours of 4:30–11pm and vary with the change of seasons. Behaviours include disorientation, restlessness, anxiety and wandering.

HOW TO HELP

The following can help to reduce your loved one's sleep problems:

- Careful management of physical health, including pain management.
- Identify and treat comorbid sleep issues, such as sleep apnoea.
- Management of caffeine and alcohol intake. If you think your loved one may be hungry at night, try a light snack just before bed or when they first wake up. Leave snacks in the room.
- A frequent need to urinate may disrupt sleep. Try to manage fluid intake in the hours before bed. Where incontinence is an issue, specialist pads will help with sleep, comfort and dignity.
- Increase physical activity and exercise in the day, preferably in natural daylight.
- Manage and minimize daytime napping if it starts to compromise night sleep.
- Increase stimulation and meaningful occupation in the day.
- Ensure there is enough relaxation time before bed.
- Routine is important, with consistent bedtime and waking times.
- Lighting is important to help your loved one's orientation. Keep it soft at night.
- Cues and prompting – putting on nightwear to communicate bedtime.
- Ensure the bedroom is quiet, reassuring, warm and relaxing.
- Medications such as melatonin can be discussed with a doctor.

REGULAR EYE, HEARING AND DENTAL CHECKS

These are critical in maintaining good health and wellbeing and to avoid unnecessary anxiety and stress in people with dementia. Poor eyesight can put someone at risk in their own home, poor hearing can increase communication difficulties and dental problems can result in a loss of appetite.

EXERCISE AND DIET

Regular exercise helps to maintain mobility and stimulate the senses and it is important to help your loved one maintain a healthy, balanced diet. Some may eat too much – and the wrong kind of foods – and some may forget to eat and drink, particularly as their dementia progresses. Supporting your loved one to keep hydrated is also essential. Missing out on essential nutrients will reduce a person's resistance to illness and can cause or increase confusion.

HOW TO HELP

To support a healthy diet:

- Take time to explore your loved one's food preferences and encourage them to be as involved as possible in food preparation.
- Consider whether the current approach to shopping and accessing meals is working well to make sure there is a regular supply of well-balanced food in the house.

- Try some simple alternatives – such as finger foods and snacks – if it seems that your loved one is not eating or drinking enough, and make these visible and accessible.
- Keep alert to any chewing and swallowing problems and seek medical advice if necessary.
- Food is often enjoyed more when in the company of other people. Try to eat together whenever possible and seek the support of other family and friends to help at mealtimes too.

ESTABLISHING A ROUTINE

Losing the ability to recognize time can lead to confusion due to a loss of structure in the day, resulting in frustration and anxiety. Establishing a routine with your loved one can help with orientation to time of day, maintain independence and increase feelings of safety and security. For example, you might help them to wake up, shower, have breakfast, do daily activities, eat lunch, rest, engage in shared interests, exercise, dinner, wind down, bedtime. Prompts and reminders such as white boards, calendars, big clocks and making the bed in the morning can all help with orientation to time. A sleep routine is particularly important.

CREATE A SAFE, FAMILIAR LIVING ENVIRONMENT

Familiarity is the key to creating a comfortable living environment. Making changes, such as rearranging the furniture, or even a new bedspread or curtains, can result in confusion and disorientation. Perceptual difficulties in dementia may result in your loved one having problems understanding their environment. Unhelpful environmental features include:

- Dim lighting
- Busy patterns on carpets, curtains, wallpaper, etc.
- Shadows and reflections
- Sudden changes in flooring (e.g., a dark or heavily patterned rug)
- Lack of contrast (e.g., toilet and toilet seat the same colour as the rest of the room)
- Too much noise or too many people

SUMMARY

Living with dementia does not need to be a barrier to living a life rich with meaning and purpose. Focus your energies on the areas that will improve your loved one's quality of life and see beyond the illness. Take time to explore and nurture what matters to your loved one in terms of their relationships, health, interests and strengths. The more you personalize your approach to their interests and lifestyle, the more everyone will benefit. Although your loved one will require increasing levels of support to maintain interests and connections to others as the dementia progresses, nurturing these opportunities will be of huge benefit to you both.

KEY POINTS TO REMEMBER

- Maintaining a good quality of life is possible following a diagnosis of dementia.
- You can do this by supporting your loved one's connections with others, helping them maintain their identity and stay in good physical health within a supportive environment.
- Connect with your loved one's strengths, qualities, and interests using the Tree of Life story approach.
- Enjoy the moments that offer opportunities for connection, and engagement in meaningful activities.

CHAPTER 5

LOOKING AFTER YOURSELF

"I have come to believe that caring for myself is not self-indulgent. Caring for myself is an act of survival."

Audre Lorde, American writer and civil rights activist

So far you have been working on accepting your loved one's dementia diagnosis and the changes this will bring to your lives. You have thought about your values and what kind of carer you want to be, and you have considered ideas to enhance your loved one's quality of life in line with your values and the principles of person-centred dementia.

This chapter is going to show you that looking after yourself is an essential part of caring for your loved one and reducing your own risk of becoming unwell. We will offer some ideas about how to do this. Many carers struggle with the idea of self-care, unsure how they could possibly add this to their 'to-do list' and believing that self-care is selfish. Does this sound like you?

As psychologists, we understand that we cannot help others in our lives and work if we neglect ourselves, although this can be challenging. As mentioned earlier, caring for a loved one with dementia is often compared to running a marathon. It requires preparation, stamina, dedication, and a willingness to open up to pain. It is important to pace yourself and ensure you are getting enough rest and recovery to cope when you feel you have 'hit the wall'. Ignoring your own health will only compromise the care that you can provide in the longer term, so it is vital that you learn to look after yourself for your loved one as well.

HOW DOES CARING AFFECT HEALTH?

Unpaid carers provide billions of pounds worth of care across the world. Without the dedication of carers like you, many of the most vulnerable people in society would miss out on vital care. According to the Alzheimer's Association (2020), when it comes to providing caregiving in dementia, it is mostly women who find themselves in full-time caring roles, shouldering the emotional and financial tolls that accompany this. Globally, two-thirds of primary dementia caregivers are female and in developing countries, this rises to nearly three-quarters. Considering women's increased risk of developing dementia alongside the risks that being a carer brings, dementia can be considered a global women's issue.[17]

The 2019 World Alzheimer Report 'Attitudes to Dementia' is the largest survey on attitudes to dementia to date. With almost 70,000 people across 155 countries and territories completing the survey, they found that:

- 75 per cent of carers say they are often stressed between caring and meeting other responsibilities, even whilst expressing positive sentiments about their role.
- Over 50 per cent of carers globally say their health has suffered because of their caring responsibilities, even whilst expressing positive sentiments about their role.
- Stress is a normal part of life and in the short-term, it can have various benefits, including boosting productivity and motivation. However, when stress becomes chronic it can negatively affect health. Whilst many carers report personal satisfaction from their caring role, research shows that carers of people with dementia are at high risk of developing depression, cardiovascular disease, insomnia, and other health-related conditions.

Adjusting to changes and the unpredictably of dementia, managing daily tasks, and role changes can all take their toll, mentally and physically. Isolation is commonly reported as many carers report being cut off from their social circles. The changing nature of the relationship may result in feelings of loss regarding your sense of companionship, intimacy, and support from a lifelong partner, further adding to isolation. Loss of self-identity can also be common due to carers having little time to engage in previous hobbies or activities.

SIGNS AND SYMPTOMS OF BURNOUT

Whilst everybody will experience stress differently, there are certain signs and symptoms to look out for. Ignoring these or hoping they will just go away will invariably make things worse in the longer term. Do any of these signs of burnout feel familiar?

Denial: 'Of course he can make himself a sandwich; he is just being stubborn.'

Irritability/short temper: 'Everyone is annoying me – I wish they would all just go away and stop bothering me.'

Anxiety: 'I feel tense most of the time. What will happen when she needs more care than I can provide?'

Low mood, feeling hopeless and resigned: 'I feel hopeless and just don't care anymore about anything.'

Exhaustion: 'I'm too tired and can't complete daily tasks.'

Difficulty sleeping: 'I can't switch off and have a never-ending to-do list. I am overwhelmed by concerns – what if she falls or leaves the house and gets lost?'

Changes in appetite: 'I am comfort-eating junk food or can't face cooking so don't bother to eat at all.'

Drinking more alcohol or misuse of prescribed or illicit substances: 'I'll just have another glass of wine to help me to relax.'
Withdrawing from social supports: 'I can't be bothered to see friends and family anymore; they don't understand anyway.'
Poor concentration: 'I have read the newspaper but can't remember what I just read.' Carers often express the concern that they must be developing dementia because of the impact of stress on concentration.
Worsening health/poor compliance with health management: 'I keep forgetting to take my medication even though I don't feel well, and have given up my daily walk.'

Please talk to your doctor if you are experiencing these symptoms on a regular basis without relief. We will now look at how you can learn to manage stress differently to reduce the chances of it becoming chronic and strengthen your resilience.

CHANGING FOR THE BETTER

'Self-care is so important and should feature regularly in our daily routine, but it is not easy, especially as we feel all that guilt. As carers, we tend not to think about our own wellbeing, only that of our loved ones, but it is extremely important to look after oneself in the first instance if we want to be able to look after our loved ones.'
Shirley

'Pain' is the unavoidable discomfort that comes into our lives when faced with difficult life events. This is no more evident than when a loved one is diagnosed with dementia. Watching the deterioration in their health and abilities is very painful and significant adjustments are required, practically and emotionally. 'Resistance' is any attempt made to avoid feeling pain e.g., denying your loved one's difficulties or using alcohol or substances to dull such feelings. 'Suffering' arises when we resist pain – it is the emotional and physical tension that we *add* to our pain. How we relate to our pain will determine how much we suffer. So, whilst it is not possible to do away with pain, we can reduce its intensity. Learning to manage painful life events involves turning toward them, accepting them for what they are and responding with understanding and kindness. Fighting reality, by holding tightly to how you think things should be or how you wish they would be, will only wear you down and compromise your ability to support your loved one. It is a bit like driving, when the car skids in a puddle; we are taught to turn into the skid, which can feel counterintuitive, but this is how we regain control of the car.

"Learning to manage painful life events involves turning into them, accepting them for what they are and responding with understanding and kindness."

BEING RESILIENT

Resilience is defined as the process of adapting well in the face of adversity, trauma, tragedy, threats or significant sources of stress. The word resilience originates from the Latin verb *resilire*, or 'to leap back' or 'to recoil'. Resilience is not a personality trait that only some people possess. On the contrary, resilience involves behaviours, thoughts, and actions that you can learn and develop by focusing on the aspects of your life that you *can* control and modify, whilst you care for your loved one. Being resilient does not mean that you will not experience emotional pain or distress, but it will help you to manage and adapt when times are tough, and to come out the other side. Like building any muscle, increasing your resilience takes time and practice. Resilience can also be drawn from other people, including other carers, who may better understand what you are going through.

Individual resilience factors (inner resources) include:

- Natural characteristics, which may be physical, emotional, and intellectual
- The ability to cope with difficult challenges
- Independence
- Social ability; having an easy temperament
- The feeling of contribution, being valuable; a sense of self-worth

- Experience of meaning and continuity; a sense of coherence and purpose
- Creativity
- Control, self-confidence, safety, awareness of self
- The ability to be of help to others and to ask for help
- Responsibility

Of note is that people do better than they anticipate in response to challenging life events. Cast your mind back to past challenges. What helped you to get through? By looking back at who or what was helpful in previous times of distress, you may discover how you can respond effectively to new difficult situations. Remind yourself of times you found strength in the past and ask yourself what you learnt from those experiences.

We will now explore some practical ideas and strategies for how you can improve your wellbeing and reduce suffering by focusing on what is within your control. Return to your values (see page 47) and use these to guide you now, in relation to your own self-care.

KNOWING YOUR LIMITS AND MANAGING EXPECTATIONS

Many carers are reluctant to ask for help. Perhaps you think that you should be able to manage things yourself. Perhaps you worry that asking for help will feel like a burden to others. You may worry that if you ask for help, people will refuse or help reluctantly, both of which can make you feel worse. You may be worried that if someone else does help, they will not understand your loved one's needs like you do, or that your loved one might become distressed without you. You may feel so tired and overwhelmed that you don't know what help you could benefit from. Guilt is often a big barrier to asking for help. Although these concerns are reasonable, it is important to acknowledge your limits and have reasonable expectations of yourself to avoid burnout. Exploring options for support for your loved one in advance, and supporting their relationships with other people, will nourish you both and give you valuable and essential time apart.

- Ask yourself what advice you would give to a friend in this situation. Our expectations are almost always higher when it comes to ourselves, so this can be a useful way to check expectations and assess how fair and realistic you are being to yourself.
- Come up with some realistic goals and do something for yourself regularly, even if it seems small. Instead of focusing on tasks that seem unachievable, ask yourself, 'What one thing can I accomplish today that helps my wellbeing?' Can you think of something small that you can do for 10–20 minutes each day? How can you build this

into your day? It is important to build in regular time away from your caring responsibilities each day.

- Just as promoting healthy lifestyle factors will help to maintain your loved one's wellbeing, so too will they help to maintain yours. It is vital that you eat well, practice good sleep hygiene and take regular exercise. In terms of supporting your health through food, extensive research points to the Mediterranean diet as having significant benefits for heart and brain health. Optimize your health by prioritizing these areas along with stress reduction, avoiding smoking and toxin exposure, and enhancing opportunities for social engagement. This will reduce your risk of heart disease, obesity, diabetes, depression and dementia.

TAKING CARE OF YOUR MIND

When things fall apart and we are faced with painful life events, difficult feelings and thoughts usually appear. Feelings of shame, anger, despair, and confusion may be familiar. You may ask yourself, 'Why has this happened to us?', or 'Why can't I cope?' You might think, 'This isn't fair,' or tell yourself, 'I'm useless.' Self-criticism is often due to the impossible standards and expectations we place on ourselves. Do any of these thoughts and feelings sound familiar? Our response to them is often to go into 'fix' mode and our instinct is to do anything to avoid feeling bad. However, no matter how hard we try to 'fix' these feelings, they reappear the next time things do not go according to plan, when new challenges arise, or when a loved one is struggling. It is just not possible to avoid feeling bad at times.

Supporting your loved one can bring up a wide range of emotions and frantic thoughts. Feelings of resentment, guilt, sadness, and anxiety are commonly experienced. Grief is also common. Coming to terms with irreversible and upsetting changes in your relationship, and role reversals, is painful. As the illness progresses, your loved one may appear to have less interest in the world in addition to a loss of shared memories. They may struggle to recognize you or other family members, which can be a source of great pain after a lengthy and intimate relationship. It is important to acknowledge these losses and let yourself grieve. You are not a bad person for having any of these feelings, and if most of us are honest, we would admit to having them too. Problems arise when such feelings are considered unacceptable and shameful. As much as we would like to not feel certain emotions, we have little control over them. The same goes for our thoughts. Whilst we cannot control our feelings or thoughts, we *do* have control over what we do and how we respond when difficulties arise.

IDENTIFYING FEELINGS

Look at all the feelings listed in the following exercise and circle all that apply in any given week. Add any other ones too. When you reflect on what you have circled, you will see that caring can certainly feel like a rollercoaster ride of emotions.

EXERCISE
Your Feelings

Keep track of your feelings from week to week by listing those that apply.

sad   happy   angry   frustrated   surprised

ashamed   embarrassed   bored   tense

jealous   tired   excited   peaceful   calm

pessimistic   optimistic   content   determined

overwhelmed   insecure   worried   frightened

guilty   lonely   tense   inadequate   lost

proud   valued   appreciated

grief   resentful   stupid   resigned

hopeless   helpless   worthless   doubtful

energetic   satisfied   loving   trapped

Learning the skills in this chapter takes a lot of practice and is an ongoing day-to-day process. Please do not give up. Just like learning a new language or taking up an instrument, it will take time to manage your thoughts and feelings differently. Changing how you respond and what you do is initially achieved by using conscious awareness and attention, which takes energy and effort. However, with time, these skills will become easier, more automatic and require less conscious effort.

Labelling your feelings has been shown to calm the brain; specifically, the amygdala – the part of the brain that sounds an alarm in times of danger. Naming how you are feeling can help to make the amygdala less active so that you feel a little calmer. This can also help to explain why we often feel better when we have talked to a friend about how we feel or written our feelings down in a diary or journal. Try to get into a routine of checking in with how you are feeling throughout the day, naming whatever feelings you are having so that this process becomes more automatic and helpful. Taking rhythmic breaths can also help to calm the autonomic nervous system.

EXERCISE
Breathing with Rhythm

When you notice you are feeling stressed, take a few minutes to pause and try the following:

1. With your shoulders, back and chest open, take a deep breath through your nose and slowly count to four. It can be helpful to count each number in your mind as you breathe, so thinking: one, two, three, four.
2. Exhale through your nose to a slow count of four.
3. Inhale – one, two, three, four.
4. Exhale – one, two, three, four.
5. Continue to breathe slowly, deeply, and evenly, in and out through your nose. If you are breathing deeply, you should naturally feel your stomach rising on the in-breath and falling on the out-breath – don't force this or worry if your stomach isn't moving. Breathing slowly and deeply is the most important thing.
6. Repeat this cycle for at least a minute. Once you feel comfortable you can then try increasing the time to five minutes or more. The key here is to breathe slowly and deeply – this has the physiological effect of slowing your heart rate and sending messages to the brain that everything is ok.

EMOTIONAL ACCEPTANCE

Central to caring for yourself is emotional acceptance – learning to see your feelings and thoughts without judgement or attempting to get rid of them. Acceptance does not mean resigning yourself or giving up, or that you must like or condone your feelings and thoughts. Rather it means opening fully to them, right here and now, without judging them or battling with them. Sometimes in our pain, we believe that the agony will last forever. However, we have about as much control over our emotions as we do the weather and, like the weather, everything you feel – anxiety, sadness, and joy – will come and go eventually. Just as we can manage different weather with aids like sunscreen and umbrellas, so too can we learn to manage difficult feelings, thoughts and sensations through the strategies outlined in this chapter. Acceptance means that you continue to move toward doing the things that really matter to you, despite having difficult thoughts, feelings, and sensations. Acceptance is having a sense of knowing everything will take its course and even in the most vulnerable states along the journey with dementia, we accept every part of our being. Acceptance can help you to be open to the various challenges that come with dementia with flexibility, and help you to readjust when necessary. Mindfulness skills offer a means to develop such acceptance.

"Acceptance means that you continue to move toward doing the things that really matter to you, despite having difficult thoughts, feelings and sensations."

Mindfulness

"Self-care and being mindful gives you permission to take care of yourself first. This helps me to see everything afresh, without judgement and worry. It allows me to experience life rather than just getting through it."
Shirley

Over the years, the practice of mindfulness has grown in popularity, but there are a lot of misconceptions about what it is and what it can do. Mindfulness is not a panacea or cure-all for the world's ills. It is not about clearing your mind of thoughts and its aim is not to make you feel better. Rather, mindfulness offers a way to reduce distress by *opening up* to pain, if there is pain to be felt, and making space for whatever difficult thoughts, feelings or sensations are coming up for us, at that time. Mindfulness is the ability to feel your pain and stay out of the drama.

Jon Kabat-Zinn, American professor of medicine and founder of Mindfulness Based Stress Reduction (MBSR), defines mindfulness as, "Paying attention in a particular way:

on purpose, in the present moment, and non-judgementally." By learning to notice what is happening in the here-and-now, we can become observers of our inner experiences without being so quick to make evaluations or judgements about them. We often live on autopilot; going through life without really being aware of what we are doing right here and now. For example, we might be having a shower or talking to a friend, but at the same time be thinking about that to-do list, what we are going to eat for lunch, what we forgot to do yesterday. So often we spend our lives ruminating on the past or getting caught up in the future, we miss out on what is right in front of us. Developing a balance between planning for the future, learning from the past and connecting with the present can help to nurture our health. Learning to be able to refocus your attention on the present is also essential when spending quality time with your loved one, so that you are connected and can make the most of this time.

"Mindfulness is the ability to feel your pain and stay out of the drama."

The skills that follow can help to cultivate mental stability and emotional awareness in the face of difficult events and situations. Instead of fighting against them, these strategies can help you to acknowledge your thoughts and feelings, no matter how painful they are, without getting hijacked by them and, instead, respond with kindness and understanding. It is important to remember that even though you may feel relaxed after practising mindfulness, that is not the goal. Sometimes the practice will be anything but relaxing, and your mind may feel busy and heavy. Instead of focusing on the outcome, focus on the process of anchoring your attention to the present moment. One simple way and quick way to start is by noticing the way you breathe.

EXERCISE
Mindful Breathing

Try this simple breathing exercise:

1. Breathe deeply, noticing how the air enters in through your nostrils and expands your lungs.
2. You can choose to focus on the warm air as it slowly exits your nostrils or mouth.
3. Pay attention to your in-breaths and out-breaths for a few minutes.
4. Remember, the mind will naturally do what it is used to doing – producing thoughts, which will divert your attention. Don't worry. Just notice that this is happening and gently bring your attention back to your breathing, as many times as needed.

DROPPING ANCHOR

Have you ever had a day when everything feels like it is going wrong, and you feel like running away? This is completely normal when you're feeling overwhelmed by strong feelings and difficult thoughts, as frequently arise within the caring role. The next time this happens, try this practical strategy called 'dropping anchor' by Dr Russ Harris, who compares breathing to an anchor. He describes how during an emotional storm, the anchor will not get rid of the storm, but it will hold you steady until the storm passes.[18] This may be in the presence of your loved one or when you are on your own. The more you practise, the more automatic and immediate its steadying effects will be. Harris encourages us to use the ACE formula.[19]

A = **Acknowledge your thoughts and feelings:** Kindly and silently acknowledge what you are experiencing internally: feelings, thoughts, physical sensations, memories, urges. Be curious about these experiences, observing them non-judgementally, as a part of you that you can notice and be aware of. While you are continuing to acknowledge your thoughts and feelings, also …

C = **Come back into your body:** Connect with your physical body. There are different ways of doing this. You can find your own way or try some of the following, doing them slowly and with focused attention:

- Push your feet hard into the floor.
- Press your fingertips together.
- Straighten your back and spine; if you are sitting, position yourself upright and forward slightly in your chair.
- Stretch your arms or neck; shrug your shoulders.
- Notice your belly rising and falling as you breathe in and out.

It is important to note that this strategy is not about distracting yourself or avoiding what is going on in your inner world. The aim is to remain aware of your thoughts, feelings and experiences and to continue to acknowledge their presence at this time. You must also come back into your body by actively moving it. This is to help you to gain control over your physical actions, even when you are unable to control your feelings. And as you acknowledge your thoughts and feelings and come back into your body, also …

E = Engage in what you're doing: Get a sense of where you are and refocus your attention on the activity that you are doing. Here are some ideas to get you started, but you can also come up with your own method:

- Look around and notice five things that you can see.
- Notice three or four things that you can hear.
- Notice what you can smell or taste.
- Notice what you are doing.
- Finish by giving your full attention to the task at hand.

When feeling overwhelmed, or if you are struggling, run through the ACE cycle slowly, with intent and focus, a few times. It can last a few minutes. It is important not to miss out the first step of acknowledging the feelings and thoughts that are present, especially if they are difficult and uncomfortable. Skipping the 'A' step will turn this strategy into a distraction technique and that is not what it is intended to be. Distraction, whilst helpful at certain times, will not help you to cope with difficult thoughts and feelings in the long run.

OLIVE AND FAITH'S STORY

Olive's mother Faith was in the moderate stages of dementia and had moved into residential care. To Olive's surprise, Faith adjusted better than expected to being in the home, which was a relief. Olive visited most days but as Faith's dementia progressed, saying goodbye at the end of the visits became increasingly fraught. Faith would get very distressed when Olive said she needed to leave. Olive's sense of guilt increased; she already felt guilty about her mother being in care. As a result, she started staying longer and longer to postpone the inevitable pain of leaving. We discussed some possible ideas to help her leave and to manage her feelings of guilt and sadness. Olive asked if a member of staff could join her and Faith in conversation about ten minutes before it was time to leave. Once engaged in an activity or conversation with the member of staff, Olive would then give Faith a kiss and hug and say goodbye, before leaving. This helped to foster a sense of security in Faith who, although still upset to see Olive go, was able to enjoy the company of the staff. We then focused on Olive's intense feelings of guilt and sadness. Once out of the home and in her car, Olive started to practise 'dropping anchor' (see page 91) for five minutes. Although these feelings never left her at the point of leaving Faith, over time Olive began to manage them without becoming so overwhelmed and distraught. This helped her to enjoy being with Faith more, rather than every visit being consumed with the dread of saying goodbye.

SELF-COMPASSION AND YOUR INNER CRITIC

In today's hyper-competitive world, our sense of worth is often attached to our accomplishments. We believe that making mistakes and messing up is something to be ashamed of, rather than simply being an expected part of life. This can result in critical self-talk – that 'voice in the back of your head' that says you are not good enough. Critical self-talk is not evidence that something is wrong with us that needs to be fixed. It is simply part of being human. Caring for your loved one can trigger such experiences daily, which if not managed, can really wear you down.

Self-compassion is essential to becoming emotionally resilient in your caring role and thriving in life more generally in the face of challenges. Self-compassion is not the same as self-care, in the superficial sense of buying yourself some flowers or doing something nice; nor is it simply being kind. Rather, compassion is best understood as turning toward distress, whether it is in yourself or others, and taking action to alleviate it. Self-compassion is a readiness to engage with pain as it arises, for whatever reason.

Professor Paul Gilbert, British clinical psychologist and founder of The Compassionate Mind Foundation, says that self-compassion is "This ability, when we are suffering, to stand back and say: 'What is this about? Why do I feel this? And what would be the most helpful thing for me now?'"[20]

No matter what, some days will just feel like a write-off. Nothing seems to go the way you want. You will feel upset and frustrated. When this happens, it is important not to beat yourself up, as this will only add to your pain and suffering. Accepting our flaws and mistakes does not mean that our behaviour cannot or should not change for the better. Rather, we can try to do things differently whilst being kind to ourselves. Learning to accept your limitations and manage the expectations you place on yourself is just as important as accepting those of your loved one. This will enable you to be a 'good enough' carer, taking the good days alongside the bad, whilst letting go of striving for perfection or drowning in despair.

EXERCISE
The Inner Critic

Notice how you talk to yourself in your head.

Is your tone kind, reassuring and encouraging or is it hostile, critical and bullying?

"Learning to accept your limitations and manage the expectations you place on yourself is just as important as accepting those of your loved one."

Just like resilience, self-compassion can be developed through practising the exercises in this chapter. Do not worry if it feels strange or difficult to begin with. Learning to give yourself a break when things go wrong is as important as valuing what you manage daily. A wealth of research shows the many benefits of self-compassion for depression and anxiety as well as for grief, trauma, and addictions. Self-compassion will help you to cope better with stress and pressure, to manage failures and setbacks, and to handle emotional or physical pain more effectively. We have discussed the power of words and how they shape our experiences for better or worse. Many of the destructive words we hear go on inside us – part of our internal mind chatter.

With all of the challenges that come with caring, the inner critic can be very strong.

It can be helpful to understand self-criticism as a dialogue between two parts of the self. There is one part of you that is critical and angry, and there is another part of you that is receiving it, feeling criticized and hurt. By seeing your inner critic as a relationship, you can step out of it and relate to the conflict in a different way. Many of us have become adept at avoiding uncomfortable or unpleasant emotions – whether it is because we are distracted by our busy lives, or simply unable to cope with what we might find, only to be blindsided when feeling overwhelmed. The first steps toward self-compassion are:

1. Gaining awareness of our inner world: what triggers feelings of anger, guilt, or sadness
2. Understanding how we instinctively react to these feelings

3. Understanding the content (and tone) of our internal dialogue, and any blocks or resistances we encounter – it is unrealistic to expect to silence our inner critic altogether

4. Directing kindness toward yourself. This can be the hardest step for many of us. It is often easier to show kindness to others. If this feels familiar, ask yourself again, what would you say to your best friend if they were in your shoes? What tone of voice would you use and what words of comfort would you say if they were feeling overwhelmed and hurt? Learning to treat yourself as you would a friend in pain will help you to start to nurture your skills of self-compassion.

"Learning to treat yourself as you would a friend in pain will help you to start to nurture your skills of self-compassion."

The inner critic thrives on stressful times, when it is most likely to be triggered. However, you can strengthen your capacity to respond with more kindness when you notice your inner critic giving you a hard time. Speaking kindly and supportively helps us to feel better. The idea is to find words that evoke tender, caring, warm feelings inside you. It is helpful to keep the phrases simple and easy to repeat – for example, 'I am doing the best that I can.'

"Be kind to yourself. It's not easy at first, but does get better, and it makes perfect sense if you stop and think what is good

for YOU beforehand. Remember to pamper yourself and do something you enjoy – perhaps socializing with friends, swimming, exercise in the park or retail therapy – whatever makes you feel good and relaxed. This will ensure your interactions with your loved one are positive, interactive, supportive, and fun. Worthwhile all round."
Shirley

This practice is an acquired skill and takes time. Many people will find it difficult or awkward to begin with. Persevere. Notice if your inner critic tells you to 'give up' or that these ideas 'are stupid or won't work' and keep trying despite such internal struggles trying to put you off. This is a practice for life as with any exercise or new skill; it is not just for when you are feeling stressed or when times are tough. Practice this each day, for a few moments, seconds, minutes or longer. In time, it will become more natural, and you will find yourself better able to manage the more challenging times.

PRIORITIZE RELATIONSHIPS OUTSIDE OF THE CARING ROLE

This is just as important for you as it is for your loved one. Connecting with empathic and understanding people is essential to prevent isolation and remind yourself that you are not alone.

Focus on finding trustworthy and supportive people who listen to you and understand your feelings. The complex feelings that can arise when caring can lead some people to isolate themselves, but it is important to accept help and support from those who care about you. It is vital that you learn to ask for help and support in order that you can create time for yourself and go the distance. Asking for help may not come easily. It is a skill that requires practice, just like the other skills in this chapter. If this seems familiar, then please make sure to put the effort into learning to ask for help so that you can take the breaks you need. The earlier you learn how to do this the better, for everyone. Whether you go on a weekly date night or meet with a friend, try to prioritize genuinely connecting with people who care about you. Spending time with only your loved one will not be good for either of you.

WHEN RELATIONSHIPS HAVE BEEN DIFFICULT

Relationships naturally go through ups and downs. When we feel disconnected from a loved one, we feel pain, sadness, loss and worry. Feelings of love can come and go, even with your nearest and dearest. You cannot control this. However, crucially, despite how you feel, you can still behave in a loving way. You may not feel like talking, but you do it anyway. You can feel angry or worried but remain calm. Drawing on your values can help in this regard. It may be that your relationship with your loved one has been fraught in the past, and this can make caring especially difficult, leading to resentment and resignation. If you have had longstanding issues in your relationship with your loved one, it may be advisable to seek further support from a professional to avoid burnout.

SUSAN AND MARGOT'S STORY

Susan reported longstanding problems in her relationship with her mother, Margot. As an only child, when Margot developed dementia Susan felt trapped and resentful, resulting in depression. She couldn't see a way out. She felt duty-bound to look after Margot but struggled with feelings of anger for her mother's parental shortcomings and unavailability. Despite her best efforts, Susan never felt she was doing a good enough job. Her resentment grew as she felt more and more unappreciated by Margot. Things were very difficult for a few years, but Susan persevered with putting into practice the different strategies she was learning to support her mother, whilst also looking after herself and acknowledging her own feelings of hurt, rejection and anger with greater acceptance. As Margot moved into the later stages of dementia, Susan noticed a shift in their relationship; for the first time in her life Susan felt connected to her mother. She spoke of their increased affection and new-found ability to hold each other's hand – something her mother had not done, even back to her childhood. Susan spoke movingly about how Margot's late stages of dementia offered a reparative, improved experience within their relationship, and that even at the end stages of dementia the possibility for something new and better arose.

CONNECTING TO OTHER CARERS AND SEEKING HELP

Although using your own resources and the kinds of strategies listed here may be enough for building your resilience, at times you may feel stuck or have difficulty making progress. Getting help when you need it is crucial in building your resilience. Having a list of dementia organizations to hand (see Useful Resources) can be a big help when it comes to getting the advice and information you need, and managing anxiety and worries. It can be extremely helpful to talk to other carers about how they look after their loved ones, and their coping mechanisms. If you are unable to meet other carers in person, you can look to connecting online. Knowing about meal delivery services, in-home help, respite services, community centres, support groups, and so on, will mean you are informed for when such supports might be needed.

SUMMARY

Learning to nurture and care for yourself emotionally, physically and socially is an essential part of managing the caring role. Despite the uncertainties and stresses that you may face, developing the skills of resilience, emotional acceptance and self-compassion will help you to manage the more difficult times, whilst also being able to value the day-to-day moments that bring you meaning and a sense of purpose. Focus your energies where you do have some control. Remember, try to treat yourself as you would your best friend, if they were going through what you are.

KEY POINTS TO REMEMBER

- Caring for yourself is an essential part of caring for your loved one.
- Take care of your body and mind. This is just as important as your loved one's health.
- Prioritize relationships outside of the caring role.
- Connect with other carers and start asking for help.

CHAPTER 6

IMPROVING COMMUNICATION

"At the end of the day people won't remember what you said or did; they will remember how you made them feel."

Maya Angelou, American poet and civil rights activist

Communication plays a critical role in relationships, at all stages. The path to developing productive, caring and supportive relationships is through good interpersonal communication. When dementia comes along, relationships and communication will change. Tom Kitwood (whom we introduced in Chapter 1) argued that communication changes associated with dementia are not fully accounted for by brain changes. Rather, changes in communication are due to the interplay between brain disease and the person's psychosocial environment. Your loved one is a 'PERSON-with-dementia' rather than a 'person-with-DEMENTIA'. Your loved one's communication with the world around them is influenced by their personal biography and character, but also their day-to-day interactions with other people, as you can see below:

- PERSON with dementia
- Family
- Community
- Wider society
- Political and economic context

There is a rich and multi-layered context around the person with dementia. Communication will vary and differ greatly depending on the context and situation that your loved one finds themselves in, and this will will influence what is communicated. For example, being surrounded by family or friends will have a different impact on how your loved one communicates compared to being in a supermarket with relative strangers. Different demands and expectations will be placed on your loved one depending on the different contexts they find themselves in. Therefore, it is important to widen your gaze and look to the world around your loved one. How your loved one expresses themselves will depend on who is around. Instead of 'managing' and 'minimizing' communication difficulties, this chapter encourages you to really think about supporting communication through consideration of language, non-verbal elements, and creative interaction with your loved one. Curiosity, creativity, and openness are incredibly important. Despite the challenges associated with dementia, your loved one will continue to seek connection within their relationships through the communication of their identity and needs, and you can support them with the ideas and strategies that follow.

FEATURES OF COMMUNICATION

True or False?
People with dementia completely lose their ability to communicate over time.

This statement is false. Personhood is made real through relationships, and central to relationships is communication. Communication is a basic human need. Yet, people with dementia are often ignored when they have something to say or there are poor attempts to engage them meaningfully; something which is required when language abilities deteriorate.

In our work, we often encounter totalistic and damning statements about how the person with dementia is 'unable to communicate'. On meeting the person, it's a different story. Often, visible changes in communication are put down to the neurological features of dementia (i.e., brain disease) with no acknowledgement of the role of psychological and social factors in supporting or limiting communication. An example of this might be that people assume that dementia stops the person expressing themselves and so they are not always involved in conversation. If your loved one is struggling to communicate, they may withdraw socially and simply give up trying. Being excluded from conversation, which may be unintentional, can lead to feelings such as depression and frustration, which will affect a person's ability to communicate further. If this seems familiar, then we need to ask several questions. Is this person being deprived of the opportunities for real communication and connection with others? Are the communication problems due to dementia, or are they socially induced?

EXERCISE
Opportunities for Real Communication

Ask yourself, is your loved one …

- Involved in discussion with family and friends?
- Encouraged to participate?
- Asked for their opinion?

- Asked to share ideas?

If speech is impaired, what alternative means of expression are used?

It is much easier to say that communication is no longer possible. We frequently hear this from professionals as well as family and friends, which places the responsibility on the person with dementia rather than the people around them. Communication is a two-way process and there needs to be flow. Remember how multilayered the context is, as discussed at the beginning of this chapter. To understand your loved one's needs and experiences, you have to try seeing their way of the world, experiencing it in their shoes, and taking contextual factors into account. This chapter will help you to do this by offering an understanding of communication in dementia, alongside tips and strategies that will enable you to remain connected to your loved one as dementia progresses, enhancing wellbeing for you both.

"To understand your loved one's needs and experiences, you have to try seeing their way of the world, experiencing it in their shoes."

Communication is something we tend to take for granted. In all, it is quite a complex process, taxing many parts of the brain and its functions. There is the sender and receiver of the message. The information then must be shared according to a common set of rules.

FEATURES OF HUMAN COMMUNICATION

- Thinking
- Listening
- Speaking
- Non-verbal

For most people with dementia, one or more of these elements may be impacted by the disease process. As you learned in Chapter 2, dementia affects functions such as memory, orientation, understanding, judgement, learning and language. However, words are far from our only means of communication. We use three components when communicating a message:

1. Words make up 7 per cent.
2. Tone and pitch of voice make up 38 per cent.
3. Body language, facial expression, posture, and gestures make up 55 per cent.

This highlights the importance of how we present ourselves to a person with dementia. When the ability to use words deteriorates, tone of voice, body language and gestures become the primary means to communicate. Central to coming to terms with your loved one having dementia, is accepting that they cannot change the way that they communicate with you. However, with the strategies and ideas outlined here, and by focusing on what is within your control, you can learn to adjust your responses and enhance your mutual sense of connection.

CHANGES IN COMMUNICATION IN DEMENTIA

"We know the feelings but don't know the plot. Your smile, your laugh and your touch are what we connect with."

Christine Bryden, person with young-onset dementia, author and advocate

First, we must consider your loved one's perspective. Losing communication abilities can be one of the most frustrating and difficult problems for people with dementia, their families, and carers. As dementia progresses, your loved one will find it increasingly difficult to express themselves clearly and to understand what others say. We have explored in earlier chapters how language and sharing stories is essential in maintaining our sense of self and identity, in the past, present and future, and within our relationships. Language makes a place for us in the world and informs how we understand and how we act. When language begins to break down, we need to become creative with communication, especially through non-verbal means.

Due to the uniqueness of each individual with dementia, difficulties with communication, expression and language will also vary. Remember that communication difficulties go beyond language and are also related to the social situation and specific skills and abilities related to this.

Some changes you might notice in your loved one include:

- Difficulties in finding words – substitutes might be offered
- Using words in the wrong way – syntax and grammar breaks down
- Making statements or asking questions repeatedly
- Speech that does not make sense – incomplete or vague statements
- An inability to understand what you are saying – in whole or in part
- Deterioration of writing and reading skills
- Loss of the normal social rules of conversation – interruptions, turn-taking
- Difficulty in expressing emotions appropriately

- Bi-lingual or multi-lingual speakers may revert to their mother tongue. Over time, the mother tongue may also endure change as outlined above.
- Progressive reduction in speech, so much so that it may finally stop altogether

SENSORY CHANGE

There is increasing awareness of the links between sensory loss and dementia. Sensory change can be more accelerated in people with dementia, and having both dementia and some form of sensory loss is common. It is important to check that communication problems are not due to impaired vision or hearing. Your loved one may need glasses or hearing aids. If they have them already, check that their hearing aids are functioning correctly and their glasses are cleaned often, as well as taking them for regular hearing and sight checks.

BEYOND WORDS

True or False?
People with dementia become more sensitive to
non-verbal communication.

This statement is true. As dementia progresses, the ability to reason and think logically will change and deteriorate.

Consequently, your loved one will increasingly rely on non-verbal cues to make sense of what is being said and, in turn, communicate their needs through feelings and behaviours. In a way, your loved one is developing new communication skills and enhanced abilities to navigate the changes they are experiencing. Even if they do not understand what is being said, they will continue to make sense of what is being communicated at an emotional level. This occurs through increased sensitivity to tone of voice, body language, facial expressions, and mood, right until the end of life. Words may fade but feelings persist, so there remain multiple opportunities for connection. Here are some ideas and strategies to support your loved one's communication.

"Words may fade but feelings persist, so there remain multiple opportunities for connection."

Listening

When we listen, we must stop talking! Talking and listening at the same time is difficult. Listening is more than being quiet. We must pay careful attention and make ourselves fully present, right then and there. Our aim is to invite the person with dementia to share their thoughts and concerns and feel safe in doing so. When we listen in a concentrated and sensitive way, we are in a strong position to tune into the person's communication style. Here are ways that you can actively listen to your loved one:

- **Be patient and slow down:** Your loved one may need time to find the right word. Let them think and speak without interrupting them. Rushing will result in stress, which will further compromise your loved one's ability to express themselves. Expressing your impatience or frustration will cause more difficulties. Self-care and being aware of your own emotional state are essential to slowing down and managing frustration.
- **Say again:** It is OK to repeat information and questions. If your loved one does not respond, wait a moment and ask again.
- **Summarize:** Repeat back what you have understood and check with them to see if you're right. Keep it short and concise.
- **Encouragement:** Reassure your loved one to take their time. This can give a confidence boost. Try saying, 'It's important for me to hear what you have to say. Just take your time.' (See 'Words of Encouragement' on page 127.)
- **Be agreeable:** Arguing with a loved one with dementia is unhelpful and counterproductive. Even if you disagree, be agreeable. What they think has happened feels real to them. Acknowledge their feelings and offer them reassurance. Also, do not point out when words or names are used incorrectly; just go with it.

- **Be creative:** If you do not understand, try guessing what your loved one is saying, or ask them to point or gesture. Focus more on the overall message than the literal words being spoken. Reading body language and emotions is important.

Voice and Speech

We have seen how much the tone and pitch of the voice contribute to communication. The voice and its quality can mean so much in connecting with your loved one. The sound is crucial. Emotion is expressed in the voice. Be aware of this. Your loved one will be able to pick up if you are feeling anxious, frustrated, or tired by the way you speak to them.

Getting caught up in your feelings and reactions will compromise your ability to effectively communicate. Looking after your own health and emotional wellbeing will help you in this regard and subsequently improve communication with your loved one. When you are stressed, speaking loudly, shouting and over-exaggerating words will distort your speech. To enable communication, do not cover your mouth as this will interfere with lip-reading. This book was written in the middle of a pandemic, when mask wearing really hampered this vital signal.

Conversation Pointers and Promoting Inclusion

Here are some ideas to help you remain verbally and socially connected to your loved one:

- Remain calm and talk in a gentle, matter-of-fact way.
- Use your loved one's name and repeat it to improve engagement. Check in with what they would like to be called and do not take this for granted. They may prefer a term of endearment.
- Depending on the type and stage of dementia, you may have to introduce yourself if your loved one has problems with recognizing people, for example, 'Dad, it's Jim, your son.'
- Keep sentences short and simple, focusing on one idea at a time.
- Always allow plenty of time for what you have said to be understood.
- When speaking about other people, use orienting names or labels such as, 'Your friend, Helen.'
- Avoid asking too many direct questions. People with dementia can become frustrated if they cannot find the answer. Ask questions one at a time, and phrase them in a way that allows for a 'yes' or 'no' answer.
- Try to avoid complicated decisions. Giving some choice is important, but too many options can be overwhelming.
- Avoid metaphors and figures of speech – for example, instead of 'tieing the knot' say 'getting married'.
- Introduce the topic and 'set the scene' for the person e.g., 'Let's talk about your brother Syed and his job.'

- If your loved one does not understand what you are saying, try to get the message across in a different way, rather than repeating it. Break down complex explanations into smaller parts and try written words, pictures or objects.
- Humour can help and may relieve the pressure. Try to laugh together about misunderstandings and mistakes where appropriate. Laugh with the person, not at the person. You know the person best to see if humour is appropriate. Gauge it carefully.

As dementia progresses, be mindful of the following:

- Include your loved one in conversations with others. Adapt the way you say things slightly. Being included in social groups will help to preserve your loved one's sense of identity and reduces feelings of exclusion and isolation.
- As dementia progresses, your loved one may become confused about what is true and not true. If they say something you know to be incorrect, try to find ways of steering the conversation around the subject rather than contradicting them directly. Arguing or trying to persuade your loved one will not work due to the cognitive changes, and will only make things worse. Pause and step back at such times. This will help to bring perspective and acceptance that their reality differs from yours. Letting go

of unhelpful battles and struggles will be one of the most effective strategies available to you.

- Try to see behind the content to the meaning or feelings your loved one is sharing.

"Letting go of unhelpful battles and struggles will be one of the most effective strategies available to you."

HOW TO HELP

Patrisha is 64 years of age and living with a rare dementia, which affects her speech articulation, thinking speed and eye movements. We asked her what would enable her to express herself more easily and she came up with the pointers below. Keep these in mind to help your loved one.

- Be patient and give us time to respond.
- Slow down when you're talking.
- If we struggle finding the word, help us out – sound it out or offer ideas.
- Use gestures.
- Read the written word when there are difficulties.
- Repetition can be annoying, so take care with this.
- Don't talk for us or talk over us.

- Don't exclude us; find a way to bring us into the chat.
- Don't move around when talking.
- Don't laugh at us.

Body Language

How often do you think about your body language? The way we hold ourselves and how we use our body conveys a great deal. Body language is non-verbal communication such as posture, gestures and the movements we make. It's just as vital as verbal communication.

- When we are stiff and rigid in our posture, it may communicate, 'I'm nervous', 'I'm feeling worried' or 'I'm frightened'.
- When the body is relaxed and movements are smooth and easy, this might say, 'I'm ready to hear' or 'I'm in a good mood'.
- When someone holds themselves strong and stands confidently, it may communicate, 'I know what I am doing' or 'I am reliable and predictable'.
- When a person nods their head, it says, 'I'm listening' and 'I'm interested'.

Every move you make with your body will convey a message to your loved one, so it is important to pay attention to how you present yourself. The reverse is also important. Pay attention to your loved one's body language before you interact. What are you noticing in them?

HOW OUR BODIES COMMUNICATE

- Eye contact
- Head movement
- Facial expression
- Gestures
- Proximity and touch
- Posture

Negative body language, such as sighs, crossed arms and raised eyebrows, can be easily picked up. Approach your loved one from the front rather than the back – this way they can see you or feel you approaching them and be more prepared for an interaction. Being approached from behind could potentially feel frightening and intimidating. Try not to stand over them and, preferably, get on their level. Paying attention to these details can help you to communicate positively with your loved one, to make yourself understood and to show you care for them.

Eye Contact: To help with quality of the interaction, making eye contact is important. The eyes are important messengers and will give your loved one the sense that you are committed to hearing them. Be careful of intensity and gaze, though. Some people find maintaining eye contact difficult, which may be related to neurological issues (eye movements are difficult), developmental issues (adults with autism spectrum disorders), or having unusual experiences (some people may be hallucinating, and so eye contact can be frightening). In getting to know your loved one's preferences, you will begin to learn their tolerance and comfort levels.

Head Movements: Using parts of the body can strengthen a message and give your loved one every chance to understand what you are trying to convey. Nodding your head up and down gives a sense of being listened to. Express agreement or disagreement by nodding 'Yes' or shaking your head 'No,' along with saying the words. This may sound obvious, but it really helps to enhance the message you are conveying.

Facial Expression: Your loved one should be able to see your face clearly, at the same level as them and straight on. A warm smile conveys a message just as strongly as words. Wearing a mask can hinder this and so other components of communication become important such as eyes, and tone and pitch of voice. Make sure that your body language and facial expression match what you are saying.

Gestures: You may need to use hand gestures to make yourself understood. Pointing or demonstrating can help. If you ask your loved one about eating something, point to the mouth or fridge to reinforce the message. If you are going out, point to clothing and the door.

Proximity and Touch: Where appropriate and with permission, use touch to hold your loved one's attention and to communicate feelings of warmth and affection. Touching and holding your loved one's hand helps with focus and conveys feelings of safety. Standing too close can feel intimidating. Instead, respect personal space and drop below eye level. This will help your loved one to feel more in control of the situation. Physical contact communicates your care and affection and can provide reassurance.

ENVIRONMENT

Think about the environment when communicating. Consider the physical environment and make sure the area is quiet and well-lit. Try to:

- Avoid competing noises, such as TV or radio.
- Have regular routines to help assist communication through predictability.
- Use visual cues. Write your message down if your loved one can read and use objects or pictures to help them understand. For example, put pictures on the kitchen cabinets, or on the door to the bathroom, or show images of what meals they can choose from.

Steps to Successful Communication in Dementia Care

Good Beginnings	Check hearing and sight Approach from the front Use person's name Get to person's level Active listening Think about feelings and meaning Introduce yourself
Facial Expression	Eye contact Smile Relax Use humour
Voice	Think about tone and pitch Tone should match your facial expressions and body language Gentle and relaxed tone
Body Language	Think about your posture, head and body Relax your shoulders, reduce your hand movements when talking Avoid sudden, quick movements Use gestures in a timely fashion

Words and Speech	Patience
	Give extra time
	Slow down your own pace
	Short and concise
	Summarize and check in
	Be inclusive
	If there is confusion, start the conversation again
Environment	Quiet and calm
	Think about routine
	Be timely
	Minimize distractions

WHAT NOT TO DO WHEN COMMUNICATING WITH YOUR LOVED ONE

It is just as important to be aware of what hinders connection due to unhelpful communication approaches. Again, keep personhood (your loved one's wishes, needs and preferences) and your values as reference points. Take care with the choice of words and the statements you use. Also, remember what Patrisha said (see page 119). The following are examples of unhelpful communication patterns:

- Steer clear of arguments with your loved one – it will only make the situation worse. Even if you know you are right, let it go.
- Avoid giving orders.
- Rather than telling your loved one what they *cannot* do, focus on what they *can* do.
- Don't talk about your loved one as if they are not there or talk to them as you would to a young child.
- Avoid condescending tones – talking down to the person may be picked up on, even if the words are not understood.
- Try not to ask a lot of direct questions that rely on a good memory.

TAKING CARE WITH WORDS

Here are some unhelpful phrases to avoid, and useful and considerate phrases to encourage your loved one to remain expressive and socially connected:[21]

What to Avoid Saying

- 'You've just asked me that.'
- 'You don't go to work anymore.'
- 'Your mum died a long time ago.'
- 'Can't you think of something to do?'
- 'You've forgotten again.'
- 'I've already told you.'
- 'Wait a minute.'
- 'Stop doing that.'

Words of Encouragement

- 'I can never remember either.'
- 'It can be hard to think of things.'
- 'Let's do this together.'
- 'I really need your help.'
- 'I'm feeling lonely and lost too.'
- 'I could do with a friend too.'
- 'Isn't it frustrating when you can't think of the word?'
- 'Is it something to do with ...?'

SUPPORTING COMMUNICATION IN THE LATER STAGES OF DEMENTIA

True or False?

People with dementia have no means to communicate in the later stages.

This is false. Despite negative narratives, it is possible to support communication right through to the end of your loved one's life. People in the most advanced stages of dementia do not lose the ability to communicate. Communication becomes important more than ever, but requires some creativity.

So, what happens when your loved one is unable to talk and appears unresponsive? A sensory approach helps in the later stages, especially engaging with touch, smells, taste and sound. Without words, you can make your loved one smile, you can soothe them when they cry and make sure they are comfortable. Sit close if appropriate so they have the best chance of hearing and seeing you. It is important to recognize that you are caring for someone who has a long life behind them and they have many stored memories and experiences. If you can connect your loved one to these memories, you can find means to communicate with them and nurture their spirit at this final stage of life. Talking in a calm, soothing voice about their past and current interests (for example, how the family are and what the children and grandchildren are doing) can offer reassurance even if the words do not appear to make sense to them. People in the late stages of dementia are often good at detecting a physical presence, maintaining an awareness of body language and remembering voices.

"It is possible to support communication right through to the end of your loved one's life."

Next, we share ideas for you to support your loved one in the advanced stages of dementia, drawing on the work of UK-based communication experts John Killick and Kate Allan.[22]

MAKING CONNECTIONS WITHOUT WORDS

If your loved one has experienced loss of language early on or when they are entering the later stages of dementia, their circle of support must work more creatively to prevent depression and anxiety. It is vital that each sense is thought about and that alternative forms of stimulation are explored to ensure connections and relationships are maintained.

Smell

Scents and smells are associated with times in a person's life and help to bring back memories of times gone by. Smelling a freshly baked loaf of bread or cake is a powerful experience for a person who enjoyed baking. Using scents such as favourite perfumes, colognes, flowers, or work-related products like oil or woodchip can remind the person of their multiple roles in their life and their achievements.

Taste

With care and perhaps with input from speech and language therapy, continue to feed your loved one orally, even when swallowing is faltering, and try stronger, sweeter flavours. Cold drinks are more easily sensed in the mouth than tepid ones. Remember to talk to your loved one about what they are eating. Offering explanations and descriptions of what you are offering is important. It is also helpful to model what they might need to do, by showing chewing motions and cutting food into small pieces.

Touch

Holding hands, massage, stroking your loved one's face, hands or arms, or brushing their hair can be soothing and pivotal in making a connection. They may like the feel of a silk scarf on their neck or the texture of wood in their hand from days of crafting. Comfort blankets, sensory cushions and rummage boxes (see Chapter 4) all offer your loved one a means to connect through touch and textures. These become particularly important when you're not around.

Doll therapy is an evidence-based intervention that can bring comfort through touch. This is especially effective should your loved one believe they are living in their early parenting years and if they appear to be seeking out children. Remember, personalizing is important. Objects and textures need to be relevant and meaningful. Connections can be made through art by holding a brush or a pencil and scribbling, finger painting, drawing on paper or moulding clay.

Sight

Think of your loved one's vision and take care with bright and dark colours. Ensure there are plenty of transfers between bed and chairs so that your loved one is not looking at the same space all day. Transfers mean that you are moving the person from one flat surface to another. Vary their view with windows and doors. If your loved one is confined to bed, place the bed by the window, if possible. Being surrounded by familiar objects is important. Family photographs, significant paintings or a favourite view can produce a reaction, perhaps encouraging them to open their eyes and reach out.

Sound

Playing or humming favourite tunes can bring back many memories; again, these need to be tailored to your loved one's life and personal preferences. Someone who lived in the countryside may react to bird song. If they lived by the coast, sounds of waves crashing on the shore may lift their spirits. We discussed the benefits of music on page 64. Often people with dementia who have stopped speaking a long time ago can sing along to a familiar tune. Depending on mobility, your loved one may connect through dancing and slow movement, which you can facilitate.

Adapted Interaction

Adapted Interaction involves communicating through sounds or movements, which can offer a means to connect in the later stages of dementia.[23] Pay attention to your loved one's behaviours and then start a 'conversation' with them, by copying or mirroring them, such as tapping a finger or pulling at a piece of fabric. You can also mirror their sighs or gentle vocalizations. Responding in ways that are familiar and meaningful to a person without speech means that a shared 'language' is being developed and this makes it possible to build and sustain close relationships.[24]

SUMMARY

This chapter has encouraged you to think around your loved one and to reflect on how communication is affected by external factors, largely social and relational. Focusing your time and energy on enabling your loved one to remain communicative will support their sense of connection to you and others. You have been introduced to considerations and strategies to look beyond the words to enable this.

"The next time you communicate with someone who is not at his or her cognitive best, remind yourself of this: 'This interaction is not about me. This interaction is about someone who is seeking connection on terms that may not advance the interests or needs of my ego. I am going to go where your needs are taking you. I am going to be with you in that place, wherever and however it is. I am going to let my ego disappear now.

I am going to love you in your image instead of trying to re-create you in mine.'"

Michael Verde, President of Memory Bridge, a US charity for people with dementia

KEY POINTS TO REMEMBER

- Communication is more than just words.
- Understand what is important to your loved one.
- As dementia progresses, your loved one will become more sensitive to body language, emotions and tone of voice.
- Enter your loved one's world by their preferred mode of communication – a shared language.
- Engaging the senses is important at all stages of dementia, but most pertinent in the later stages.

CHAPTER 7

_____

BEHAVIOURS THAT CHALLENGE US

"The person is not the problem, the problem is the problem."

Michael White, Australian family and narrative therapist

"Sometimes if he was in a bad mood while I was upstairs showering and dressing him, he would say that he didn't want to speak to me. We would carry on in silence. After he went downstairs, I would finish getting myself ready. Then when I came down looking a bit different, I would say brightly, 'Good morning Robert, and how are you today?' He would look a bit confused. I would keep on talking to him, and he would assume that I was the 'other' Edna. This would ensure that we had a nice, peaceful day and it put his mind at rest."

Edna

As Edna's experience shows, sometimes we need to take preventative measures, based on the needs of our loved ones, to reduce their distress. In this chapter, we share some ideas and strategies to help you do that. We will help you to identify common triggers for behavioural distress and we outline the how the world around the person with dementia can feed into behaviour. We will also return to the principles of person-centred care (see Chapter 1), so you can be equipped to respond to and meet your loved one's needs. It is all about being a detective and taking control of what you have control over!

UNDERSTANDING BEHAVIOUR CHANGES

True or False?

People with dementia deliberately misbehave to wind others up.

This statement is false. People with dementia have increasing difficulties communicating, including saying if something is hurting or distressing them. The way that they behave at these times may be labelled and viewed as 'challenging' by other people. Poor handling of such behaviour can result in more emotional distress, for you as well as for your loved one. There is a particular sensitivity in the use of language here. We use the term 'behaviours that challenge' as opposed to 'challenging behaviour'. The term 'behaviours that challenge' pays respect to the complexity that surrounds your loved one and that behaviours are related to both personal and external factors (e.g., personality, family structure and support, accommodation etc.). In contrast, 'challenging behaviour' locates the blame and responsibility in the person with dementia with little reference to what might be going on around them. In this chapter, we discuss a range of behaviours that can feel challenging for carers – from unusual experiences, verbal and physical acting out, to withdrawal and pacing.

Behaviours that challenge bring difficult emotions to those who are caring. Seeing your loved one constantly pacing can be distressing as you realize that it gets in the way of eating and relaxing. You may start to feel defeated, thinking, 'This is hopeless' and 'I'm helpless to make a change here.' This may result in feelings of anger, anxiety and depression and illustrates how distressed behaviours in dementia become the carer's challenge.

RESPONDING TO DISTRESSING BEHAVIOURS

A 'critical point' must be passed when an action is regarded as challenging, which entails a judgement by others.[25] It is important to be aware of biases and the tendency to make judgements prematurely when distressing behaviours emerge. Remember Social GRRAACCEESS on page 10? Be careful of jumping to conclusions and be aware of your own biases and the power of difference. What is challenging to one person may be different for another. Try to remind yourself that your loved one's thinking and memory processes that govern behaviour are breaking down due to the disease processes.

One of the most significant mistakes is to see the behaviour as intentional. If your loved one's behaviour is distressing and out of character, then they are *feeling* distressed. They are not behaving like this for fun or pleasure. Telling yourself, 'Mum is doing it on purpose' is very different to telling yourself, 'The dementia can sometimes affect mum's behaviour and communication'. Changing your perspective to the latter offers you the best chance of remaining empathic and responding in more helpful ways. The way we respond to a situation depends on how we make sense of it and how it makes us feel. Behaviours do not emerge in isolation. In this chapter, we will show you how to reframe behaviours by building on the context around the person. Remember, all behaviours are understandable at some level.

"Try to remind yourself that your loved one's thinking and memory processes that govern behaviour are breaking down due to the disease processes."

COMMUNICATION OF UNMET NEEDS

True or False?
Behaviours that challenge in dementia are an attempt to communicate an unmet need.

This statement is true. The key understanding here is that all behaviour is a form of communication, and behaviours that challenge are your loved one's attempt *to* communicate an unmet need in the only way they can.[26] We discussed in the last chapter how your loved one will increasingly communicate through their feelings and behaviours as dementia progresses. Arguably, they are attempting to be resourceful and creative given their cognitive limitations. This chapter is all about identifying your loved one's needs and trying to meet them to prevent distress. Although many people with dementia will display behaviours that challenge at some point, behavioural disturbance is not an inevitable consequence of dementia.

Furthermore, the occurrence of behaviours that challenge can be reduced significantly and, with better understandings and responses, be eliminated entirely for some people.

"Behaviours that challenge are your loved one's attempt to communicate an unmet need in the only way they can."

WILLIAM AND AUDREY'S STORY

William and Audrey have been married for 50 years. William has dementia, but overall is physically fit. Audrey is living with complex physical health. They continue to live together in their home. In the earlier stages, William felt frustrated and angry. There were times when he would shout, swear and, on occasion, push Audrey. She would argue back and then began to take over many of the household tasks. She said it was for an easier life. Meanwhile, William would sit there, often on his own and brooding.

William was communicating through his behaviour that he was bored and lacking a sense of purpose or role in the house. Due to his deteriorating language abilities, he was unable to communicate this verbally. What we see as frustrated, sometimes frightening, behaviour was his way of telling others what his needs were: 'I need something to do and to occupy myself with.' When Audrey was encouraged to share the household chores with William, the behaviours reduced. As soon as he started vacuuming, going to the corner shop for milk, and painting the woodwork in the garden, William began to feel calmer and more relaxed. He felt a sense of purpose and that he was contributing to the relationship again. Audrey had thought that she was doing a good thing by not overloading William with things to do, but it had left him bored and feeling useless.

IDENTIFYING FEELINGS

Your loved one will continue to experience the same feelings as you. However, changes in their thinking and memory, along with increasing changes in communication, will mean they increasingly struggle to express these feelings. For this reason, changes in behaviour can be an indication of a feeling. We need to look beyond the actual words or actions and search for the underlying feeling being communicated. If, for example, your loved one says, 'I want my mum' or 'I want to go home', they may be communicating the need for security and love. Ignoring or diverting them by telling them, 'You are at home' or 'Your mum died years ago' will not address the underlying feelings being expressed.

HOW TO HELP

It is important to take time to try to understand the meaning behind your loved one's feelings to better meet their needs and improve wellbeing and feelings of safety.

- **Depression:** Sadness, loneliness, worthless, negative, hopeless
- **Anger:** Loss, grief, rights infringement, protection of self-esteem, pride
- **Fear:** Vulnerability, exposed, chaotic, unpredictability
- **Shame:** Dignity breached, dependency, faults others are aware of, humiliation
- **Disgust:** Lack of control, dependency on others, failure, shame
- **Contempt:** Actions or judgement from others as being worthless
- **Happiness:** High self-esteem, strong sense of identity, acknowledgment and appreciation, contentment
- **Pride:** Well connected to skills and talents, sense of purpose and achievement

As you may experience, more than one behaviour can be present at a time. Ian James, a British psychologist in dementia, differentiates between two types of behaviours:[27]

1. **Non-active forms of behaviour** include withdrawal, apathy and depression.

2. **Active forms of behaviour** include reactions to stressful situations: excessive walking and pacing; interfering activities (e.g., packing belongings, emptying cupboards), difficulties in 'following through' and 'inhibiting' actions (e.g., abandoning tasks, swearing), and mismatching between the person and the environment (e.g., a person being in a boring environment when they have always been so active).

HOW TO HELP

Recall a time when your loved one showed signs of distressed behaviour. In a notebook or journal, make a list of the behaviours you observed and experienced.

Now ask yourself:

- Is the behaviour really a problem?
- What is my loved one trying to tell me?
- Why in this way?
- What needs are not being met?
- How can I meet their needs?
- Who finds the behaviour problematic?
- What external factors might be aggravating them?
- Are there any safety concerns?

TRIGGERS AND CAUSES OF DISTRESSED BEHAVIOUR

Generally, distressed behaviour may represent:

- An attempt to meet a need (e.g., to sleep, to seek company).
- A signal that there is a current unmet need (e.g., pain, boredom).
- To communicate frustration (e.g., a carer helping too much and taking over).
- The person's experience of the world is challenging to them (e.g., misperceiving shapes).[28]

When your loved one is expressing distress, the situation must be assessed thoroughly so that you can try to help them. It can be useful to think of the distressed behaviours as the 'tip of the iceberg' – see the image opposite.[29] Above the line (the surface or tip) is what can be observed in the person; a range of behaviours and emotion. Below the surface of the iceberg lie the 'hidden' but relevant factors that influence your loved one's behaviour and feelings. These are influences we cannot see. In William's case (see page 140), underlying his shouting, pushing and swearing (the 'tip') lay boredom, a sense of redundancy and a lack of purpose.

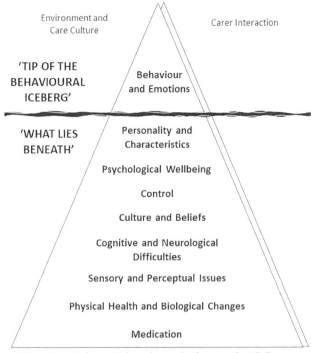

The Iceberg Analogy to Help Understand Behaviours that Challenge
Adapted from James & Hope, 2013

THE TIP OF THE ICEBERG – WHAT'S VISIBLE

True or False?

*Distressed behaviour may be due to a combination
of multiple factors, including physical, environmental
and interpersonal.*

This statement is true. Before we explore further what lies beneath distressed behaviour, it is important to evaluate your loved one's environment, the care culture and their interaction with other people. Remember, social and environmental factors will affect your loved one positively and negatively.

HOW TO HELP

Consider these aspects of the care environment:

- **Physical:** How is the lighting, noise, temperature, stimulation?
- **Social:** Are there opportunities to be with different people or is your loved one isolated?
- **Cultural:** Does your loved one have access to features of culture and heritage – occasions, rituals, expression such as art, music, poetry, conversation?
- **Emotional:** Does your loved one experience validation, empathy, acceptance, attention and opportunities for meaningful communication with others?
- **Spiritual:** Does your loved one have access to people of faith and spirituality (e.g., cleric, priest, leader etc.)? Have they access to a place of worship? Are they encouraged to practice and express their spiritual or religious views and practices? How frequent is this?

Now consider the care approach adopted by you and others. Are there inconsistencies and different approaches in how your loved one is supported? Is it person-centred? Is the person's voice heard? As discussed earlier in the book, becoming a carer is not a role many people have planned for. Perceptions and responses to stress in dementia will differ from person to person. Also, different people in your loved one's life will have different levels of tolerance for change, uncertainty and distress. What is deemed challenging by one person may not be experienced as such by another. A close family member is likely to have a different emotional response to that of a paid carer who did not know the person previously. Remember that your loved one will become increasingly sensitive to body language and your emotional responses. Your interactions can act to alleviate or exacerbate emotional distress through your responses and approach. Self-care, and having an awareness of yourself in the moment, will be important in how you manage and respond to any behaviours that challenge you.

"Self-care, and having an awareness of yourself in the moment, will be important in how you manage and respond to any behaviours that challenge you."

WHAT LIES BENEATH – THE HIDDEN FACTORS

Going back to the iceberg analogy (see page 145), it is important to pay attention to your loved one's psychological wellbeing, physical health, and consider social and environmental factors. Issues in any of these areas can result in them becoming distressed. Paying attention to these areas will help you to make sense of what your loved one is trying to tell you through their behaviour, and may reveal solutions to meet their needs.

Personality and Characteristics

The starting point is to connect to your loved one's life history, character and personality. This can help to improve your bond more generally when problems feel overwhelming, but also offers clues as to the meaning of certain behaviours. Working together on a life story or Tree of Life review (see page 57) will help with this.

Psychological Wellbeing

Anger, worry and sadness are basic human emotions, universally and cross-culturally. This is no different for your loved one. Mood changes are common in dementia and may be expressed through behavioural disturbance. Key signs of mood changes may include your loved one appearing sad, more withdrawn and less interested in doing activities they used to enjoy, along with low energy, poor sleep and changes in appetite. Or they may be more confused or agitated. Looking at what is going on around your loved one will help you to understand their emotional changes and find ways to help where required. Anxiety can increase when the environment is chaotic and the future is unpredictable. Anger often occurs when we feel our rights are being infringed or violated. Sadness and low mood are often associated with losses of any kind, including loss of role and purpose.

Control

We all need to have a sense of control in our lives and to feel safe and secure. Given the changes that come with dementia and increased dependence on others, loss of control is a common experience. Supporting your loved one to achieve a sense of control within their lives will help to reduce the risk of behavioural disturbance and improve their wellbeing. This might include encouraging them to have a choice about what they wear, what they eat and where they might want to go. Consulting your loved one and asking their opinion about important matters is incredibly important; especially wishes, dreams and ambitions.

SHIRLEY AND EILEEN'S STORY

Shirley has been supporting her 96-year-old mother Eileen, who is living with Alzheimer's Disease. In Eileen's care home care plan, Shirley has requested that Eileen has choices about what she wears and the food she eats. The carers give Eileen a choice of two outfits each morning and Shirley brings her an array of finger foods. Shirley explained that it is important for her mother to look good, given she always took pride in co-ordinating her wardrobe and how she looked. Shirley also asks the carers to help her mother to be independent in feeding herself – to use her cutlery and fingers for as long as possible.

Culture and Beliefs

Cultural awareness involves the recognition and respect of characteristics that make your loved one and those around them, including you, diverse. It is important to understand how cultural awareness can help with the interpretation of behaviours and the ability to access appropriate and timely attention and care. This includes the consideration of the person's country of origin, family and cultural background, preferred language, education, religion, belief system and socio-political view. Responses to behaviours that challenge can be influenced by cultural factors. Beliefs and thoughts influence how people feel and experience their world – be careful to not misconstrue what might be a religious belief with an unusual sensory or perceptual experience. For example, some people might see a deceased family member soon after they die, believing they are coming back with a message from the afterlife. This is more about grief than hallucinating. Religion remains a powerful influence on notions of health and disease as well as phenomena in dementia. We have supported families who have perceived the change in a person's thinking and memory as a spirit possession and an indication of 'badness' or poor faith. These beliefs bring shame and fear. Some people have belief systems that do not approve of different aspects of health care e.g., medication, or care approaches such as having help from outside the family. Cultural awareness will vary greatly, especially amongst those outside a family system, including friends, professionals and services. Educating others may be necessary to get the best help and to prevent misunderstandings. This might involve sharing information about the person's country of origin and its history and practices, or a religious practice or ritual.

The inner world of people with dementia is often neglected and what they do express is all too often explained away as 'confusion', 'nonsense' and 'incoherence'. However, focusing on the belief often holds the key to understanding the person's current view of their reality. Your loved one may believe they are younger and so must collect the children from school, or will talk about needing to 'go home' due to the belief that they live in a house from many years ago. Consider the impact of these factors on your understanding and care so that you can respond to your loved one's needs. Be curious and identify gaps in your knowledge; broaden your perspectives around dementia.

Cognitive and Neurological Difficulties

The nature of your loved one's cognitive changes and stage of dementia will affect their behaviour. Dementia damages different areas of the brain, which may directly impact behaviour and communication (see Chapter 6). Having dementia will also affect your loved one's ability to deal with daily stresses and increase their susceptibility to environmental stressors, which can result in distressed behaviour.

Sensory and Perceptual Issues

We experience the world through the five senses – touch, taste, smell, sound and sight. With age, our vision and hearing changes over time. Think of a time when your ears were blocked or when you may have had to wear a blindfold. How did you feel? Typically, having a sense compromised can result in confusion and disorientation. Now, think of your loved one who not only has memory and thinking problems, but may also have some sensory and perceptual changes. Keep in mind how frightening the world around them must be.

Brain changes can often bring sensory impairment. This is the way the nervous system receives, organizes and understands information from within the body and the physical environment. As such, your loved one will see the world differently and will engage accordingly. The five senses will work differently, which may lead to thought processes and behaviours that could come across as unusual. For example:

- Shadows or darkly lit areas can be difficult to figure out.
- Forms and patterns can be misinterpreted as something that is frightening and threatening.
- Touch is something that changes with age, especially sensitivity to touch and temperature. Along with brain change comes skin changes, and the person's perception of being touched will feel different. For example, some people with dementia are so sensitive to touch that a gentle pat may be perceived as a slap.
- The experience of taste may change and the person's relationship to food may be affected. Appetite may also

be complicated by mood, should someone feel sad and depressed. Taste may also be affected by medications which are taken.

"Think of your loved one who not only has memory and thinking problems, but may also have some sensory and perceptual changes. Keep in mind how frightening the world around them must be."

HOW TO HELP

You know your loved one the best. In your observations, what have you noticed about their senses? Have various senses changed over time? Be curious and ask your loved one. With their agreement and some explanations, carefully experiment by testing their senses with a variety of smells, textures, foods; all to inform your understanding and approach. Their responses will give you a good indication. Do they grimace, try to cover their ears, smile, lick their lips?

Smell: Does your loved one experience both pleasant and unpleasant scents the same? What is their reaction?

Taste: Does food taste the same? Do they still like their favourite foods?

Sound: What level can your loved one hear or not hear? What happens when there is background noise or volume changes? At what level do they hear best? What are the most conducive circumstances?

Touch: What is your loved one's experience of touch and with levels of intensity? What are the most preferred or least liked textures e.g., soft, hard, smooth?

Sight: What is your loved one's vision like in artificial light versus natural light? What happens when there is a pattern or when the environment is visually busy?

Physical Health and Biological Changes

Changes in your loved one's health can trigger distressed behaviours. Often, knowing the physical origin can help with resolving the issue. However, it may not always be easy to know if they are physically unwell as they may not be able to say what they are feeling or explain their symptoms. Being a detective is essential as it is important to rule out underlying causes. A visit to the doctor may be part of this. Illnesses such as urinary tract infections (painful urination or needing to go often), chest infections including pneumonia (chesty cough), gastrointestinal infection (tummy upset) or fever (high temperature) can lead to confusion and agitation. Skin breaks and pressure sores can also be a source of potential infection. It can be a 'double whammy'; more confusion and disorientation than you are used to. Simple checks such as blood screens, urine samples and temperature gauges can inform the assessment.

Delirium: Although delirium is often mistaken for worsening dementia, it is usually due to an infection resulting in acute confusion. If there is a sudden change in your loved one's mental state over a few hours or days, they may have an infection. They may appear confused only to seem their normal selves at other times. People with delirium typically have difficulty paying attention to what is going on around them. Thinking is more disorganized, along with agitation or increased drowsiness. Your loved one should be assessed by a doctor as soon as possible. See page 218 for a delirium checklist to become more familiar with how this presents, and on page 220 there is a troubleshooting guide, which outlines the similarities and differences between delirium, dementia and depression.

Ongoing illnesses: Conditions such as angina, heart problems, diabetes or pain associated with arthritis, ulcers or headaches, can affect a person's behaviour and mood – so it is important to ensure they are being monitored and treated effectively.

Dental issues: These can be a great source of pain, so dental and gum health should be checked regularly.

Dehydration: Many people with dementia can no longer recognize when they are thirsty, or they forget to drink, which means dehydration is common. Signs of this include increased confusion, dizziness, dry or flushed skin, fever and a rapid pulse. Prompt your loved one to drink and leave drinks out for them as a visual reminder. Set reminders if necessary.

Constipation: This is caused by a lack of dietary fibre or fluids, not enough exercise or reduced mobility. Some medications can cause constipation. Regular bowel movements are important as constipation brings significant discomfort and pain. This in turn can lead to increased confusion, restlessness and agitation. Make sure your loved one's diet contains enough fibre and fruit. Discuss with a healthcare practitioner if concerned. Try to be active together as physical activity and movement will help with bowel movements.

MARIE'S STORY

Marie has Alzheimer's dementia. She is often restless and paces for hours up and down the hallway and stairs. Being so active means little time for hydration, but Marie gets comfort from movement as she is prone to constipation. Constipation and dehydration alone can cause confusion. Add this to the dementia. Therefore, the pacing behaviour is more than just 'the dementia' and solutions were offered with regards to improving hydration and constipation, which helped.

Disrupted sleep: Sleep naturally changes with age and as discussed earlier in the book, dementia can often cause further sleep disturbance as the sleep/wake cycle goes out of sync, leading to restless, agitated behaviour. Sticking to some kind of sleep routine is important. If you notice your loved one sleeping a lot during the day and being more awake at night, try to restrict day sleeping gradually. See the sleep strategies on page 68.

Medication: It is important to ensure your loved one is taking medication as prescribed, but also that regular medical reviews are carried out, especially when they are taking multiple medications. Discuss issues related to multiple medication interactions or side-effects that may affect behaviour, with your healthcare provider.

Medication should only be considered for behaviours that challenge, when:

1. Other approaches have had limited success.
2. Behavioural symptoms are putting the person, or others, at risk of imminent harm.
3. There is distress for the person (e.g., hallucinations) or there is a medical reason underlying the behaviour (e.g., infection).

It is also important to note that medications are not effective for the following behaviours:

- Wandering
- Being unsociable
- Poor self-care
- Restlessness
- Nervousness
- Sexual disinhibition
- Sundowning (see page 170)
- Impaired memory
- Being uncooperative
- Inattention
- Verbal expressions or swearing
- Fidgeting
- Hoarding

BEING THE DETECTIVE: BEHAVIOURAL CHARTS

The previous section encouraged you to use the iceberg checklist to consider the many factors underlying your loved one's feelings and behaviours. This will help you to make sense of what they are communicating and then meet their needs when they are distressed. With time against you and so much to do, it can be tempting to jump to possible solutions. However, being a detective requires you to STOP, LOOK and LISTEN to identify what might be underlying your loved one's behaviour.

ABC ASSESSMENT

You can identify what might be underlying the behaviour by doing an 'ABC' assessment:

- **Antecedent:** What happens *before* or in the lead-up to the behaviour?
- **Behaviour:** What happens *during* the episode?
- **Consequences:** What happens *afterwards*?

Reviewing completed ABC charts can provide some answers, through better understanding and enhanced empathy around the causes of distressed behaviour. Most importantly, ABC charts can give us clues and ideas about how to help. The aims of carrying out an ABC analysis are:

- Gives you time to reflect and consider what is happening before, during and after a period of distress
- Helps you to focus on the emotion your loved one may be experiencing
- Helps you to understand what your loved one might be thinking and what they are trying to communicate
- Considers all possible clues in the environment that may be triggering or maintaining distress
- Records and monitors the duration and frequency of distress and monitors any improvements

To further enhance the effectiveness of the ABC approach, use it consistently and approach the behaviour in the same way – use the same analysis every time you encounter a specific behaviour.

On the next page, you will find an example of a completed chart. For ABC charts to be effective, it is important that you are specific about the behaviour you want to analyse. For example, we often see 'aggression' written on record forms as the 'behaviour', but what does this mean? The more clearly you define the problem, the more likely you will find an effective course of action. Set the scene and think about the context, such as the environment or the activity at hand e.g., 'noisy room', 'personal care'. Consequences are dependent on the interpretation and reaction to the behaviour; remember to check in with assumptions and bias (see page 10). The charts should only include observations – not personal judgements and opinion. Try not to guess 'why', as this comes later.

AFTER ABC COMES D

We also add D – Decide (come up with as many ideas as you can; it doesn't matter how silly they seem), De-escalate, De-compress, Debrief and Deep breathing. Ask yourself what changes you need to make. Remember the iceberg (see page 145) and consider the environmental, physical and interpersonal factors as well as making reference to your loved one's personality. How can you change A to better manage B?

Date and Time	Description	De-escalate/ Debrief Ideas/ Reflections
Antecedent/Trigger ***Ask:*** - Where was the person? - How did they present? - What day and time was it? - What was going on around the person? - Who was present? - Who was not present?	Think of the iceberg here. Consider environment, emotions, control, physical health, cognitive impairment, life history etc. Example: DON'T WRITE: *Charles was in a challenging mood.* DO WRITE: *Charles woke up several times the night before and complained of feeling tired this morning. In a snappy tone, he told me and Gill (our daughter) 'Leave me alone!' when he was asked to get dressed.*	Example: *Morning times are generally difficult for Charles. He was never a morning person before dementia and was always so grumpy.*

Behaviour	DON'T WRITE: *Charles lost his temper.*	Example:
Ask:		*Gill's presence may have been too much when I made this request. I may have been standing too close to Charles. Maybe I shouldn't have spoken to him.*
- Where did it occur?	DO WRITE: *Charles began to raise his voice and said 'Go away!', when I asked him to calm down. He left the kitchen and swore at me. Charles looked angry. He punched my right arm once and kicked the kitchen chair twice.*	
- What were the circumstances?		
- What did the person do?		
- Did they seem aware of their actions?		
- Did they appear frightened, agitated, distressed or indifferent?		
Consequences	DON'T WRITE: *Charles was told off for what he did.*	Example:
Ask:		*I should have tried to handle it myself as Gill may have made things worse.*
- What was the response of others to the person?	DO WRITE: *My arm was painful and throbbing. I got a fright. The chair was turned over. I cried out and Gill (our daughter) came to tell him he should not do these things and explained why. She said that I was only trying to help.*	
- What was said to them and in what tone? Was touch used?		
- How did you try to reduce the distress?		
- Did the person attract the attention of others for the behaviour?		
- If so, what was their reaction to the attention of others?		

Use the example table as a template and keep a log of your workings. Patterns – along with solutions and ideas – will emerge, which will then be evidence of what is or isn't helping. Share with others who provide care, if needed.

PERSON-CENTRED RESPONSES

Once you have carried out a thoughtful and considerate analysis of your loved one's behaviour, you will have a better understanding of their distress. This will then help you to develop person-centred, meaningful and individualized strategies in response. The primary aim is to prevent your loved one becoming distressed in the first place, and this should always be a priority. The relationship experience is key to a successful intervention. The responses of others are of key importance in keeping people with dementia in our shared world.

"The primary aim is to prevent your loved one becoming distressed in the first place, and this should always be a priority."

Here is a list of key features of a person-centred approach to dementia care and behaviours that challenge, many of which will be familiar if you have followed the ideas in previous chapters:

- **Don't argue:** This will only make the situation worse.
- **Respect:** Treat your loved one how you would like to be treated.
- **Basic needs:** Check if your loved one is hungry or thirsty, ask or observe if they are cold or tired and establish whether they need the bathroom. Always rule out pain and make sure there is adequate pain relief.
- **Reassure:** Actively listen to, respond and reassure your loved one. Use their name. Say, 'I know you're anxious [name], and I'm here.'
- **Communication:** Speak in a calm and gentle manner, keep it short and simple, avoid jargon, avoid rushing and be aware of your facial expressions. Smile and nod to show you are listening. Say your name and who you are if there's confusion. Check sensory needs. Can your loved one hear and see you?
- **Choice and independence:** Ensure that there is some control and choice in your loved one's life, from eating to wearing clothing and going out to visit places.
- **Inclusivity:** Choose your language carefully. Say 'we' rather than 'you' or 'I'. It is important to give your loved one a sense of control and to help them to feel involved and included, rather than doing things to them.
- **Environment:** Identify and reduce environmental triggers and safety hazards.
- **Distraction and diversion:** This can be a quick and useful strategy. With good judgement, an appropriate distraction

or activity may diffuse a situation effectively. However, be careful that you don't disregard what your loved one is saying or doing, along with how they are feeling. For example, if a person is shouting, putting a mindful colouring book in front of them is not useful when they need attention, reassurance and comfort first and foremost.

- **Stimulation with purpose and meaning:** Make sure your loved one has regular opportunities to engage in purposeful and meaningful activity.
- **Humour:** Although it can have many benefits, be careful with humour and laughter as you do not want to negate your loved one's lived experience of cognitive impairment and loss. Laugh *with* them and not *at* them.
- **Celebrate exceptions:** If your loved one overcomes distress, a fear or a worry, celebrate it. If they make the smallest of progress, acknowledge it and communicate it as an achievement. Praise and encourage those moments.
- **Psychological needs:** We have seen how your loved one will increasingly come to rely on other people to support the fulfilment of their needs. Their psychological needs are no different. Tom Kitwood developed the idea of the Needs Flower, which can be a helpful reference for you to meet your loved one's psychological needs with your behavioural interventions.[30]

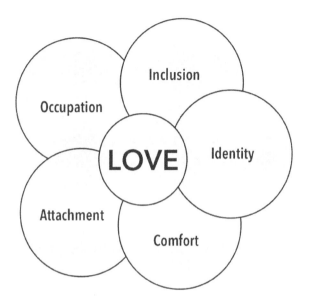

Kitwood's Flower

LET'S GET SPECIFIC – FOCUSED BEHAVIOURAL STRATEGIES

For all strategies, please hold in mind the overarching principles already introduced in this chapter. Bear in mind that behaviour that is agitated or aggressive may need additional support. If there are safety or risk concerns, speak to a healthcare professional.

Next, you will be introduced to the kind of behaviour, alongside the meaning behind the feeling. Some idea of the psychology behind the behaviour is offered. Once a sense of understanding is gained, solutions and ideas are introduced.

If several attempts have been made to ease your loved one's distress and it continues, seek additional specialist help and support. Increasing and prolonged distress, along with signs of carer burnout, are worrying and require professional assessment and intervention. Asking for help early means that there is every chance to address the behaviours that challenge.

Agitation

What it looks like: Restlessness; fiddling and vocalizations, such as talking constantly; repeating words, questions and phrases; crying and screaming.

Potential cause: Events or factors in the environment e.g., taking a bath, having flu.

Words of comfort: 'I see that you are restless. What can I do?'

Strategies:

- Remain calm; create a relaxing environment – e.g., play soothing music.
- Reduce demands on your loved one, but enable them to make worthy contributions.
- Ensure your loved one is comfortable.

- Listen to the content of the vocalization. Look beyond the words as your loved one may be seeking reassurance. Try responding to the repetitive questioning.
- Include activity and exercise regularly in your loved one's daily routine to burn excessive energy.
- Reduce caffeine or use decaffeinated beverages.
- Involve your loved one in everyday tasks so that they have a sense of purpose and control.
- Replace repetitive movements by engaging your loved one to use their hands – e.g., pairing socks, folding clothes, tearing up paper, sanding or dusting.
- When your loved one becomes stuck on one task, touching or pointing may help cue the next step.

Pacing/Wandering

What it looks like: Walking at length; following and tracking backwards and forwards.

Potential cause: Disorientation in a new or even in a familiar environment; memory and thinking problems causing confusion. Your loved one may also want to escape from a noisy or busy environment. This behaviour may also be related to having excessive energy, or your loved one may be looking for something or someone.

Words of comfort: 'Where are you going, [name]? Can I come along? Let's go into the garden.'

Strategies:

- Keep the environment clutter-free and safe. Remove any trip hazards.
- Remove triggers and objects that might encourage wandering (e.g., coats, handbags).
- Identify and record patterns of movement – e.g., times of the day.
- Feature regular walks and exercise in your loved one's routine.
- Designate a safe place for your loved one to mobilize, such as a garden space.
- Ensure your loved one has identification if they are prone to going out; place contact details in their pocket, wallet or purse. Identity bracelets and a GPS should be considered.
- Involve neighbours and local business owners. Most people are very helpful once they understand the situation, and may offer to keep a friendly eye on your loved one.

Sundowning

What it looks like: Restlessness and increasing confusion or changed behaviours in a person with dementia that occurs late in the afternoon or early evening/dusk time.

Potential cause: Body clock changes can occur in dementia and adjustment to light changes like dusk can be difficult. This causes a biological mix-up between night and day.

Words of comfort: 'It's getting late and the light is changing; let's get cosy.'

Strategies:

- Keep your loved one busy at twilight – when the light changes the most.
- Keep your loved one calm and preoccupied – e.g., ask them to help prepare dinner or set the table. Play soothing music.
- Close the curtains and keep the environment brightly lit.
- Increase exposure to natural light earlier in the day. If your loved one cannot go outside, they might sit by a window. Exposure to natural light can help reset the body clock.
- Encourage a short nap at this time (less than 45 minutes), if fatigue or exhaustion is making sundowning worse.
- Try not to arrange effortful tasks, such as having a bath, around this time.
- If the sleep-wake cycle is beginning to reverse and you and your loved one are feeling exhausted, speak to your doctor.

Aggression

What it looks like: Verbal outbursts or physically hitting out.

Potential cause: Feelings of fear, threat, intimidation or a loss of control. Potential triggers include pain, fatigue, discomfort, over-stimulating surrounds, too many questions, difficult tasks, strangers, failure at simple tasks, or confrontation.

Words of comfort: 'I know you are feeling worried. I'm here to help you. What would you like to happen?'

Strategies:

- Watch for warning signs, e.g., increased body tension or strained facial expressions.
- Avoid confrontation; try not to be critical or show irritation. Stay calm.
- Take note of what is being said – it may be a communication of need, such as privacy. For example, 'Get out!' may have been triggered by someone entering the room without knocking. (Always ask permission.)
- Keep your tone of voice low and soft.
- Say things in positive terms. Saying 'No' or using commands increases resistance.
- If there is any confusion, say your name. Also, use your loved one's name.
- Do not make sudden movements.
- Give your loved one plenty of personal space.

- Suggest a simple activity, such as having a drink together, going for a walk or looking at a magazine.
- With physical outbursts, give your loved one space and time to recover quietly. It can take 45–90 minutes for physiological arousal to return to normal levels.
- Make sure your loved one is left safely and in a dignified way. Check carefully at intervals.
- If your loved one hits out, and you've got to get close, give them ample room and clear, short explanations about what you're doing. Position your body safely.
- Get your loved one to hold something soft like a stress ball, a soft toy or cushion. It also becomes a distraction should you need to get close.

Difficulties during Personal Care

What it looks like: Tearfulness; screaming; avoidance; physical or verbal aggression, or a combination of these.

Potential cause: Becoming naked and having intimate care can be experienced as exposing, violating and a breach of privacy and dignity. It's further complicated if the person has experienced sexual abuse in their past. Confusion and not recognizing people may result in your loved one being more distressed, because it feels like a complete stranger is tending to their personal care. Feelings of worry and stress may emerge.

Words of comfort: 'Let's get you ready for the day. I'm going to run the bath.' 'I will take off your nightdress and then will help you in the bath.'

Strategies:

- Always ask permission on entering the room, on using touch and before proceeding with personal hygiene.
- Ensure it's an unrushed and consistent routine.
- Spend time explaining what is happening, step-by-step, in simple sentences with calm tones.
- Explore washing preferences – e.g., shower, bath or sink. This may need to vary depending on how your loved one is feeling both in terms of their mood and their energy.
- Pay attention to touch and textures – e.g., a hard towel may feel painful compared to a soft sponge. Ask about preferences.
- Think about temperature. Check that the water feels OK for your loved one. Make sure it's warm when they get out of the bath or shower. Heat the towel on the radiator.
- Encourage your loved one to do as much as they can, such as washing their hair or washing body parts. Use their favourite scents. Make it manageable by applying soap and shampoo on the sponge or flannel. Give simple instructions.
- Create a relaxed environment by playing calm and gentle music in the background.

Hallucinations

What it looks like: Responding to stimuli, such as sounds and visions, which others cannot hear, see or feel. This might include hearing voices, noises, seeing people or having a sensation of something crawling on their skin.

Potential cause: Feelings of fear, threat and intimidation. With the brain changes that come with dementia, processing sensory information can be difficult.

Words of comfort: 'I know you are scared. I'm here for you.'

Strategies:

- Try to respond to the underlying feeling, which is often fear.
- Don't argue or challenge unusual experiences. Try not to reason, given the heightened level of distress along with the cognitive impairment.
- Don't laugh and joke about the hallucinations. Listen and make the person feel heard.
- Avoid asking your loved one for too many details as this may bring the unusual experience to life and it makes it harder for them to forget.
- Have your loved one's eyesight, hearing and skin checked so that there is no physical underlying cause for changes in processing and perception.
- Environmentally, make sure there is enough light. Reduce glare, patterns and shadows to prevent misinterpretation

of forms and shapes. Make use of night lights but be mindful of the shadows they create.

- Encourage your loved one to talk – this reduces the intrusiveness or even stops the voices.
- Play music or put the radio on as this can reduce the frequency of auditory hallucinations.
- After acknowledging the emotion, attempt to distract your loved one. Concentrating on something other than the voices and visions will often help to obscure them. Distractions may include household chores, music, exercise, activities, conversations with friends and looking at old photos. Make sure your loved one takes interest in or enjoys the activity.

Unusual Beliefs and Suspicious Thinking

What it looks like: Strange and fixed ideas and beliefs that are not based on reality, but which are thought to be true, e.g., paranoid thinking, suspicion, beliefs about being stolen from.

Potential cause: Feelings of fear, threat and intimidation, along with problems with memory and thinking, all caused by brain changes, make this very real to the person.

Words of comfort: 'I'm here with you. I know you are frightened. You are safe.'

Strategies:

- Put yourself in your loved one's shoes. Imagine you believed that someone was out to get you and you had to live your life in fear.
- Acknowledge the emotion that goes with the unusual belief.
- Don't scold and criticize your loved one for saying unusual things or losing objects or hiding things.
- Investigate suspicions to check their accuracy. There may be a reality basis, e.g., a paid carer stealing a watch.
- Try to maintain a familiar environment to bring a sense of safety and certainty. If your loved one has to move, take some familiar things with them.
- Try to find common hiding places, but don't expose where they are as your loved one will feel upset and violated.
- Keeping a diary may help to establish whether these behaviours occur at particular times of the day or with particular people. Identifying such causes may help you to make changes to overcome the difficulties.
- If possible, keep a spare set of things that are often mislaid, such as keys, a purse or glasses.
- Some hallucinations and false ideas can be supported if they are harmless and do not cause your loved to become agitated. If they cause distress, seek professional help.
- Do not take the accusations personally, and be aware that your loved one is not able to control this behaviour.

Sexual Inappropriateness or Disinhibition

What it looks like: Actions that seem tactless, rude or even offensive, such as swearing... but there may also be sexualized behaviours such as exposing themselves, being sexualized in behavior (e.g., masturbating) or commentary.

Potential cause: Often the person is anxious and needs reassurance. Your loved one may have forgotten the usual social rules about what is appropriate to say or do. They may have forgotten where they are, how to dress, the importance of being dressed, where the bathroom is and how to use it; they may have confused the identity of a person; they may be feeling too hot or cold or their clothes may be too tight or itchy; they may be confused about the time of day and what they should be doing. Remember, a person with dementia is still a sexual person and due to the breakdown in cognition, sexual expression becomes difficult so they resort to the only ways they can.

Words of comfort: 'I'm here with you. Let's go somewhere private.'

Strategies:

- Be patient and gentle. Try not to overreact, even though the behaviours may be very embarrassing. Remember that they are part of the dementia.
- Check with a doctor whether there may be a physical illness, undesirable side-effects of medication or discomfort e.g., skin irritation.

- Give your loved one plenty of appropriate physical contact, such as stroking, hugging and rubbing to bring ease and reassurance. Take care with this as it can feed into sexualized behaviours.
- If your loved one is engaging in inappropriate sexual behaviours, gently remind them that the behaviour is inappropriate. Lead them to a private place or try to distract them by giving them something else to do, or something else to fidget with.
- Your loved one may need to be supported with regards to how to express themselves sexually. Having intimate time on their own and/or with their partner may need to be thought about sensitively, but also broadly and creatively. Consent and permission are essential every step of the way.

EDNA AND BOB'S STORY

Despite many challenges related to Bob's hallucinations and beliefs, Edna maintained a truly person-centred approach to his care and problem-solving. In the late stages of dementia, Bob believed that there were 'multiple Ednas'; good and bad. Edna was initially unsure about how to respond, but over time, she began to connect to Bob's internal world by focusing on his feelings. Edna became incredibly creative and reassuring in her responses, seeing how confused and distressing these experiences were for him. She told us, *'Sometimes he would tell me how the "upstairs Edna" wasn't very nice to him that morning. I would listen and very delicately defend her, saying, "I think she has a lot of problems at home as her husband isn't a well man and she still manages to come here to help us out even though she hasn't had much sleep."* He would then feel very sorry for her and would apologize to her. *I often thought, if I wrote a book, I would call it 'Upstairs Downstairs'."* Edna also realized the importance of self-compassion and looking after herself; she'd get through these challenges by spending time with her daughter.

"Remember that their experiences, no matter how odd they may seem to you, are their reality."

Hallucinations in dementia, such as seeing things or hearing voices and noises that others cannot, are often regarded as behaviours that challenge. The underlying emotion is often fear and worry. It is important to listen and hear what your loved one says about unusual experiences. Remember that their experiences, no matter how odd they may seem to you, are their reality. Listening and hearing will not only enhance your understanding, but it may also result in ideas to comfort and reassure your loved one.

SUMMARY

You have amazing potential to devise and implement sensitive and thoughtful strategies to cope with difficult times, with your loved one at the centre of your care. Remember that all behaviour is a form of communication and your detective skills will be needed when making sense of your loved one's unmet needs, if they present with distressed behaviours. One size does not fit all and what works one day may not work the next. Being flexible and adaptable, and drawing on your resilience and values, will help you to cope. As with all new skills, implementing the ideas in this chapter will take time, patience and practice. Remember, self-care is essential, and keep an eye out for your inner critic. Keep trying and your confidence will grow.

KEY POINTS TO REMEMBER

- When your loved one is showing distress, they are communicating unmet needs.
- There are common types, causes and triggers for distressed behaviour. Use the iceberg analogy to help you to understand.

- The ABCD approach can help to make sense of the circumstances surrounding behaviours and offer ideas for how to meet your loved one's needs.
- The most effective strategies are person-centred, individually tailored and flexible.
- When nothing seems to work, take a pause and seek help if needed.

CHAPTER 8

TRANSITIONS IN DEMENTIA – NAVIGATING THE JOURNEY

"We walk this rollercoaster of life together. We are adjusting our dance steps to the changing melody of dementia."

Christine Bryden, person with young-onset dementia, author and advocate

As you well know, life is full of transitions, where destabilization arises and results in a level of change. Some changes are subtle, with others being major and noticeable. Some are joyful while others are painful. Some transitions can be expected and planned for, whereas others are sudden and drastic. Although everyone experiences transitions and change, the way we navigate them will differ. As we have alluded to throughout the book, we refer to dementia as a journey and we use this metaphor strongly in this chapter. Supporting your loved one with dementia will mean that your voyage together will be unique, with some diversions and bumps along the way. To navigate the dementia journey, it is important to have a sense of what lies ahead and to use the information you have to manage the challenges that can arise.

We hope the previous chapters have equipped you well with ideas and strategies that get you ready to manage the difficult times, and the knowledge of when to ask for help.

It can be reassuring to have a 'journey map' and a sense of what change might look like. This can offer you a sense of control and power to shape and inform change at points of transition. Again, the focus is providing person-centred care and creating a quality of life at all stages of change in dementia. Your loved one may have an advance decision plan (see page 215), which will assist you on the journey and help family negotiate transitions successfully. This chapter introduces you to the kinds of transitions you might want to prepare for in looking after your loved one. We realize that this can feel frightening. It is important to say now that you should take your time with the content of this chapter. There is no obligation to read it in full. We have structured it purposefully, to cater for all stages and a readiness to face each stage. Every person's journey is unique.

THE JOURNEY SO FAR

Before you read on any further, what has your journey been like to date? In the exercise below, we ask you to think about the themes, your values, the lessons learnt along the way and to anticipate what might lie ahead. Write the answers somewhere you can access them readily.

EXERCISE
Think of your Journey to Date

Describe the journey[31] with your loved one since they developed dementia: (Exercise is based on ideas by Ncube-Mlilo.)

- What themes have emerged?
- Where did the journey start?
- Where are you headed to?
- Who have been the significant people along the way? Who helps? What will help will you receive from others? What will help will you give to others?
- What are the things that have kept you strong?
- What values have influenced you?
- What have been the lessons learned along the way?
- What skills will you use to travel further?
- What steps do you need to take to achieve the goals you have set?

- What do you want the world to know about you on this journey?
- What skills, abilities and knowledge can help with the challenges ahead in your journey with your loved one?

This exercise encourages you to connect to your strengths and resilience and to redress the balance, especially when you hit a bump on the road. We want you to be able to think about what works well alongside the challenges. We also hope that this kind of exercise can strengthen you to face the 'storms of life' (exercise is based on ideas by Ncube[32]) as it encourages solutions and asks you to think about building your circle of support. Restructuring family systems, entering new roles and building new lines of support may need to occur during transitions. A change will be required in the level of care and/or support required for your loved one given the known progression of dementia.

Reading this book may feel like a journey. You have been taken through an array of topics and ideas to enable you to look after yourself, whilst looking after your loved one. All, in a way, are to do with transitions.

- Recognizing the signs of dementia and getting diagnosed entails a series of typical and highly likely transitions.

- Coming to terms with the news is another important point of change. This can create instability, which leads to the creation of needs and another potential transition such as becoming a carer and finding your way with this role.
- Tending to self-care is also an important adjustment.
- With the progression of dementia unfolding, more concrete and major changes unfold.
- In the face of deterioration, care of your loved one will potentially necessitate the involvement of other people and systems like formal carers, hospitals and care homes.

Here, we coin the phrase 'the river of life'. This is our way to outline broadly, the points of change and transition with the dementia journey.

It is important to realize what point of the journey you are at. To make transitions bearable, and as smooth as possible, you need to be at the same stage together – and moving forward. Trying to maintain wellbeing for you and your loved one throughout the transitions will depend on a delicate balance of perceived need, risk and likelihood of resolution of each part of the journey.

The next sections will focus on more formal systems of support to enable you to look after your loved one. You

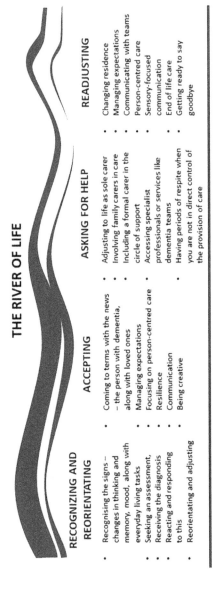

THE RIVER OF LIFE

RECOGNIZING AND REORIENTATING

- Recognising the signs – changes in thinking and memory, mood, along with everyday living tasks
- Seeking an assessment,
- Receiving the diagnosis
- Reacting and responding to this
- Reorientating and adjusting

ACCEPTING

- Coming to terms with the news – the person with dementia, along with loved ones
- Managing expectations
- Focusing on person-centred care
- Resilience
- Communication
- Being creative

ASKING FOR HELP

- Adjusting to life as sole carer
- Involving family carers in care
- Including a formal carer in the circle of support
- Accessing specialist professionals or services like dementia teams
- Having periods of respite when you are not in direct control of the provision of care

READJUSTING

- Changing residence
- Managing expectations
- Communicating with teams
- Person-centred care
- Sensory-focused communication
- End of life care
- Getting ready to say goodbye

will always be connected, albeit in a different way, with the involvement of others. This includes formal carers, respite options, care homes and end of life care. You will be introduced to some considerations with each approach and how you might negotiate these transition points.

THE JOURNEY AHEAD

"Due to a fall that resulted in a broken arm, I became unable to look after myself or Bob. He appeared to resent me for this, likely due to his fear and struggles to understand what was going on, leading to multiple threats to hit me, even whilst I tried to sleep. My last and only option left was to call the emergency services, as his behaviour was becoming increasingly unsettled and unpredictable.

I phoned and told them I didn't know what to do anymore. They took Bob away for a mental health assessment and I decided for my own wellbeing that it was time for him to go to a permanent nursing home. I was reluctant to do this, but at 83 years of age, it was taking its toll on me."
Edna

Edna's pain – and the difficulty deciding about Bob's care – is evident. Her health changed, which meant her capacity to care for Bob changed.

In the early stages of the dementia journey, depending on the carer's knowledge and personal previous experience with dementia, they might have high hopes and expectations. People often tell us that they hope desperately that everyday living tasks will be minimally affected and that having formal care arrangements or their loved one ending up in long-term care will not be an option. Hopes and expectations may require adjustment given the reality and the emotional challenges that many face. Expectations about what will happen influence how transitions occur and how quickly you adjust. Preparation before, during and after is key to making changes more bearable.

> "Hopes and expectations may require adjustment given the reality and the emotional challenges that many face."

FORMAL CARE PROVISION

Conversations about formal care and advance care planning can be difficult. They often come with difficult feelings such as guilt, shame, loss, grief and a sense of failure. These are expected and understandable feelings given the enormity of these decisions. However, a delay in recognizing and learning about your loved one's needs (e.g., day centre or respite care) can result in a delay in accessing services that may help. This also means that both of you become affected, in terms of having a quality of life and maintaining good standards of wellbeing. Remember what you learned about acceptance in Chapter 5. It is important to accept that the level of support required for your loved one is changing. Depending on where you live, these options may be available:

- Day centre or social clubs for people with dementia
- Sitting or befriending services
- Formal carers in the home
- Respite services

The options available to you will have financial implications and support arrangements can be informal, and publicly or privately funded. It is important to check statutory entitlements for your loved one as well as for yourself – for example, you may be entitled to a formal carer's assessment. This will vary considerably depending on where you live, so seek out relevant local guidance.

When making decisions about formal care arrangements, you may want to consider specific factors of the care provision:

- High-quality, flexible, responsive and person-centred care is key. Whatever your choice, your loved one's sense of self and individuality, along with a sense of control and choice, needs to be maintained.

- A personalized approach to keeping the person busy is important. Activities should have some meaning to the person and give them a sense of purpose and satisfaction while working the brain.
- For you to be most relaxed, staff need to be kind, trustworthy and knowledgeable.

"It is important to accept that the level of support required for your loved one is changing."

- Good communication should be open between your loved one, family, care staff and management. Although sometimes difficult, continuity and consistency of staffing is essential for your loved one to develop comfort and trust.
- Choice of gender of staff for intimate care may also be a point of discussion.
- Exploring respite options (i.e., you having regular breaks) keeps the arrangement at home more guaranteed and sustainable.
- It is also important to consider emergency care in instances of carer sickness.

"Life with formal carers is much easier. It takes the pressure off and helps me maintain my routine. That's so important. My carer is important to me as she keeps me at home and independent. Here is what you should expect from a carer who is entering into the home of a person living with dementia. They should:

- *Get to know us – sharing a life story book can be helpful*
- *Learn about the dementia – I have a rare type*
- *Treat us with dignity and respect*
- *Respect our privacy*
- *Give us independence and confidence – don't do everything and take over, as this causes chaos*
- *Ask for permission and involve us*
- *Try to be flexible*
- *Make time for pleasurable and fun tasks"*

Patrisha

PERMANENT CARE AWAY FROM HOME

Behavioural issues, an increasing dependency on others, safety concerns and/or complex physical healthcare needs may inform the consideration of care away from home. These decisions can be difficult to navigate when different members of the family hold different opinions and views on your loved one's needs, and can result in tension and disagreements within families, adding extra stress. Again, self-care and having open conversations about risk and needs are required. 24-hour care options may come in the form of a residential or nursing home, a specialist placement for people with dementia with complex needs, or hospital care. There may be age limits with some care provision, such as long-term care for people living with young-onset dementia. Avail of support from professionals when making these decisions.

A Care Plan

You may worry that you have no input or influence over your loved one's care, but you do. Your say becomes important now more than ever, and continued support from family and friends is key to your loved one's quality of life. This becomes formalized in the care plan: a structured summary of your loved one's care needs and preferences and how these are met through a team of formal carers. The more you can share about your loved one, the better. A life story or the Tree of Life (see page 57) can really help to tailor person-centred care. The care plan will also contain a risk assessment that seeks to minimize difficulties. A feature of such risk is understanding that there can be deprivations of liberty, such as a locked door to the premises. This is often a requirement to keep those in specialist care settings safe, especially when mental capacity is reduced.

"You may worry that you have no input or influence over your loved one's care, but you do."

HOW TO HELP

Here are some ways to settle your loved one into a home away from home:

- A period of respite beforehand may gauge your loved one's opinion and feeling for the place. If not possible, visits may help in the lead-up.
- Give time and space for staff to get to know your loved one. Visiting too much in the early phase of settling in can disrupt the formation of relationships.
- Sharing a life story with the staff can help them get to know your loved one. It also communicates preferences and gives ideas for activities and stimulation. Food preferences, how to comfort your loved one and ways to approach personal care are important points to communicate.

- Add familiar and homely touches to your loved one's room. This may include photos, pictures, ornaments, blankets, etc. Involve your loved one in making these choices. This will help develop feelings of connectedness and belonging to the surrounds. It will also help boost your loved one's sense of security.
- Support your loved one to attend the activities in the care home, and then step back.

Difficult Emotions

Adjusting to new surroundings will take time, from weeks to months. This response is individual and understandable given what a major transition it is for both of you. Your loved one's reaction can range from being relieved and content to being agitated and sad. You may be surprised at how easily they settle, or not. Some people may express their feelings by saying things about their family and/or the staff and they may plead for help or to go home. This is quite difficult to witness, but your loved one is being cared for by professionals who can soothe and reassure them. This can trigger feelings of guilt in carers (remember how Olive used 'dropping anchor' to manage her feelings of guilt when leaving her mother Faith on page 93). There are no right or wrong feelings. Some carers may have guilt put upon them by other family members or friends.

"The guilt we go through is a rollercoaster of emotions and we even start to believe we are selfish and could do better for our loved ones. These are normal feelings. It's so common to feel guilty and emotional when having to make a care home placement decision, but it's through love and care that this decision must be made. The guilt can become unbearable, but we must be positive and strong, remembering that the home can offer care and equipment that we cannot provide ourselves for whatever reason. Remember, there are so many ways to remain connected with our loved ones."
Shirley

Keep in mind that you have made this decision carefully and eventually you will be freed up to focus your energy on having quality time with your loved one. Upon hearing, 'I want to go home', it's best to reassure your loved one that they will be safe, and remind them of your love for them. This longing for home may be expressed at your departure. Take something to do. Once you have finished this, it is time to go. Let your loved one know at the beginning of the visit how long you can stay and why you have to leave. Shirley often told her mother, 'I can stay for an hour but then I have to go shopping.' Keep farewells brief and leave straight away. Lingering, apologizing or staying a little longer can make saying goodbye even harder. Ask staff to help refocus your loved one's attention to another subject such as reminiscing about childhood or family memories, or get them involved in a purposeful activity such as walking or preparing the dining room for supper.

True or False?

I stop caring when my loved one is placed in permanent care.

This statement is false. However, many carers believe that permanent care will remove them from the caring role. You do not stop caring just because you no longer do the physical tasks of caring. Allowing others to take responsibility for the practical caring tasks does not lessen the importance of your role as a carer. In fact, you are the 'expert' when it comes to caring for the person with dementia. A good care setting will honour and utilize your expertise. Here is Shirley's advice for caring from a distance:

- It is so important for us to choose the right home and ask as many questions as we can.
- Prior to any care home placement, a specialist assessment will be carried out to see what your loved one's care needs are – either nursing or residential care.
- Research costs and whether there are public or private funding implications.

- Family or friends should be consulted to help choose the option they believe is most suitable for their loved one's needs.
- Make visits to gain a true picture of how the care home is managed and operates, especially during mealtimes and activity events.
- You can contribute to personal care plans and how your loved one will be looked after.
- Ask when doctors, opticians, nurses, dentists, chiropodists etc. visit.
- Enquire about personal living space, mealtimes and menus, planned indoor and outdoor activities, garden space and visiting times.
- Make notes of any questions you have and write them down.
- When your loved one makes the move, build relationships with staff and management. Complement the good work so it encourages more.
- If difficulties arise, speak with care unit leads and management. Escalate to registration bodies if you are not happy with local resolution.
- Self-care is so important and should feature regularly in our daily routine, but it is not easy, especially as we feel guilty that our loved ones are now living in a care home.
- Join the residents' carer support group, if available.

Spending Time Together in a Home Away from Home

Some adjustment and creativity may be required when spending time together and doing activities given possible constraints in the care environment, be it a nursing or residential home or a more specialist unit for people with dementia. Again, your approach needs to be personalized and meaningful to your loved one – as the dementia may have progressed, make sure that there are not too many demands placed on them. You may also need to consult with the staff in order for some of the activities to be realized. Here is a list of ideas:

- Bring newspapers and magazines to look at together.
- Listen to favourite music or sing together.
- Make a shopping list together of what is needed, such as toiletries and snacks.
- Make decisions together about new clothes.
- Play games that have been enjoyed in the past.
- Arrange to have lunch or afternoon tea together.
- Watch a well-loved film or family video recordings.
- Look at photo albums together.
- Help decorate and tidy the room.
- Help with personal grooming – washing or brushing hair, trimming a beard, painting nails.

- Assist with writing to friends and relatives.
- Have an outing together. Try a short drive in the car, perhaps stopping for afternoon tea or lunch, visit family or friends (if your loved one can tolerate this) or take a stroll or wheel around the garden.
- Resource boxes: as well as life story books, some care homes may consider making use of resource boxes, which can be filled with items that can be used during visits to trigger conversations or ease communication between residents and visitors. This could include photographs, postcards of tourist attractions, music tapes or CDs, videos of particular events, and even things like hand creams or other sensory material like fabrics. These can be inexpensive to put together and could encourage visitors to get involved.

HOW TO HELP

Remember the suggestions made on pages 129–131 about how to use as many of the senses as possible – sight, taste, smell, hearing and touch – all to get a positive response from your loved one? With this in mind, when you visit, consider doing the following:

- A gentle kiss or hand-holding may be reassuring and comforting. A smile, a comforting gaze or a look of affection may provide reassurance.

- Massaging legs, hands and feet with scented creams or oils may be enjoyable for some people. The scent of perfumes and cologne or flowers may also be enjoyed.
- Playing your loved one's favourite music or singing to them may provide comfort and familiarity.
- Listening to a favourite book or poem being read may be enjoyable.
- A stroll around the grounds, taking in the sights and scents of different surroundings, is also something that is likely to be appreciated.

END OF LIFE CARE

"How lucky was I to be there. The care staff said Mum waited for me. I felt like she did. I held her and I said all I wanted to say. I thanked her for everything she did for me. I said I would miss visiting her and I was heartbroken that she was leaving me. I said she will always be in my heart and she will be with me forever. I said that all the family were waiting for her and she must go. I cuddled Mum into my chest and held her until her final breath. My Queen."
Shirley

In the final stages of dementia, despite the best care, your loved one is approaching the end of their life. Now, the focus is on comfort and making the most of the time that is left. Depending on their personal circumstances and whether they have other health conditions, your loved one's final stage may last from weeks or months to several years and you may find it uniquely challenging due to grief combined with ongoing daily care and complex end-of-life decisions. It is important to draw on the skills and understanding you have developed during your caregiving journey to help you through this final stage.

> "This stage of caring requires plenty of support, both practical and emotional, as you come to terms with letting go."

Conflicting feelings, from worry to sorrow, denial and anger, relief to guilt, are all common. Whatever you may be experiencing, this stage of caring requires plenty of support, both practical and emotional, as you come to terms with letting go. Although this can be an extremely painful time, the extended journey of caring can offer the opportunity to prepare for – and find meaning at – the end of your loved one's life. While this will not limit painful feelings of loss and grief, having an opportunity to express your love and say goodbye, resolve differences and forgive grudges can also help you come to terms with your loss and make the transition from caring and grief toward acceptance and adjustment.

The principles of person-centred care are just as important at the end of life. Good end-of-life care will help you to support your loved one to live as well as possible until they die, and to die well, or as they would have wished. It supports all aspects of their wellbeing:

- Physical needs (including pain relief and management of other symptoms)
- Emotional needs
- Relationships with others
- Spiritual beliefs and needs
- Environmental needs

If you are clear about your loved one's preferences in the final stages of life, you can then devote your energy to care and compassion. One of the most critical aspects to good end-of-life care is communication and information-sharing. The end-of-life journey is eased considerably when conversations regarding placement, treatment and end-of-life wishes are held as early as possible.

- Return to your loved one's advance directive, if one was made.
- Consider hospice and palliative care services, spiritual practice, and memorial traditions before they are needed.
- If your loved one did not prepare a living will or advance directive, return to their values. Act on what you know or feel their wishes and values are.

- Make a list of conversations and events that illustrate their views.
- As far as possible, consider treatment, placement, and decisions about dying from their personal vantage point.

MEANINGFUL CONNECTIONS

Even in the end stages of dementia, your loved one has the capacity to feel frightened or at peace, loved or lonely, and sad or secure. Regardless of where they are being cared for – at home, in a hospital, or at a hospice facility – the most helpful interventions are those that ease pain and discomfort. It is very important to provide the chance for them to experience meaningful connections to family and loved ones. Go back to Kitwood's flower (see page 167) to look at how to meet your loved one's psychological needs. Even when they cannot speak or smile, their need for companionship remains. They may no longer recognize you, but can still draw comfort from your touch or the sound of your voice. Remember to talk as if they can hear. Speak calmly to help reorient your loved one. Gently remind them of the time, date, and people who are with them. This will help to create a soothing atmosphere. Plan visits and activities for times when they are most alert. Return to Chapter 6 for communication tips at this stage. Reassure your loved one that you will honour their wishes, even if you do not agree with them. If children have been involved in the care of your loved one, make efforts to include them in age-appropriate ways.

If you wonder what to say to your loved one, US based palliative care physician Ira Byock, identifies the things dying people most want to hear from family and friends:[33]

- 'Please forgive me.'
- 'I forgive you.'
- 'Thank you.'
- 'I love you.'

"They may no longer recognize you, but can still draw comfort from your touch or the sound of your voice."

MANAGING PAIN

Pain is one of the most common symptoms that people with dementia experience. Even in the last stages, your loved one can communicate discomfort and pain and managing it requires daily monitoring and reassessment of their subtle non-verbal signals.

Here are some signs that your loved one may be in pain:

- **Vocalizations:** Whimpering, groaning, crying
- **Facial expressions:** Looking tense, frowning, grimacing

- **Changes in body language:** Fidgeting, rocking, guarding part of the body
- **Behavioural changes:** Increased confusion, refusing to eat
- **Bodily changes:** Raised temperature, pulse rate or blood pressure, perspiring, flushing or pallor, skin changes

Communicating such changes to the medical team is important to ensure your loved one receives the right treatment.

HOW TO HELP

There are ways to ease your loved one's physical discomfort:

- Keep them as clean, dry and comfortable as possible.
- Use an air mattress and air cushions to help to relieve pressure.
- Ensure good mouthcare and oral hygiene remain a priority.
- Breathing may be easier if your loved one is turned on their side and pillows are placed beneath their head and behind their back. A cool mist humidifier may also help.
- You can also help to ease discomfort through touch, massage, music, fragrance, and your soothing voice. Experiment with different approaches and observe your loved one's reactions.

EATING AND DRINKING

In the last few months or weeks of life, it will be natural for your loved one's food and fluid intake to decrease. Do not worry too much at this stage about giving them a balanced diet. Ensure they are fully awake and in a good position when they are being helped with taking in food or fluids. As dementia progresses, it affects the area of the brain that controls swallowing, and this can be extremely distressing to witness. Other problems – such as having a sore mouth or sensitive teeth – can cause a person to take in less food or develop swallowing problems. Bring these difficulties to the attention of your health professional. Oral fluids may be restricted in the final days due to the risk of fluids entering the lungs resulting in pain and discomfort. Mouthcare is important to make sure your loved one doesn't feel thirsty.

FINAL SIGNS

If your loved one becomes restless, report it to their doctor or nurse immediately. Restlessness could be due to pain or a high temperature and needs to be relieved.

As death approaches, your loved one's breathing pattern can change as a natural part of the process of dying. There may be periods where they are breathing regularly, then stop breathing for a few seconds. Breathing usually gets faster and there can be long gaps in between. It can sound wet or gurgling. Your loved one will be unaware of this, but it can be distressing to witness.

Your loved one's skin may become quite pale and clammy. Their fingers and feet may have a blue tinge because their blood flow is slowing down as death approaches.

Give regular mouth care. This can be done hourly to prevent the person's mouth from becoming dry. Apply petroleum jelly to keep lips moist. Gentle wiping of the eyes with a soft piece of wet, clean gauze can help with eye care.

"Reassuring your loved one it is OK to die can help both of you through this process."

Most people wish to die with family nearby, but others might prefer to go privately. Keeping a vigil can be a sacred experience and gives your loved one strength and comfort if this has been their preference. Sit with them, hold their hand and talk to them. Remember, however, that your constant physical presence is not required. It remains as important as ever to take breaks, nourish yourself, and accept support from others. Also, understand that you might not be at your loved one's side when they die. This timing is beyond your control. Some people die gently and tranquilly, while others seem to fight it. Reassuring your loved one it is OK to die can help both of you through this process.

After your loved one has died, you may draw comfort from taking some time to say your last goodbyes, talking or praying before proceeding with final arrangements. Give yourself time and go at your own pace.

COPING AFTER A DEATH

Grieving is a very personal and individual experience. You may have a mixture of feelings, from shock and numbness to relief, anger and guilt. It is normal for grief to come in waves and feel overwhelming at times. It does not mean that you will not be able to function for the rest of your life.

After your loved one dies, you might question whether you did enough or said the right things. Guilt is a normal part of grieving, but it often gradually fades.

Attend to any rituals associated with death and loss including a funeral, wake, religious ceremonies, marking anniversaries and so forth that are meaningful for you.

You may find it takes a long time to come to terms with your loved one's death. Those who have been full-time carers for a long time may be left with a huge void when this role ends. It may take time to re-establish your sense of identity. Giving yourself permission to find new meaning and relationships can be difficult, but you have earned health and happiness. Carers' bereavement support groups and grief specialists can help if needed.

Take time to reflect on your loved one's life and remember the quality time that you were able to share together. Remember that your acts of love, care and connection have sustained your loved one through this journey. Sharing what you have learned, cultivating happiness, and finding new meaning can provide a fitting finale to your caregiving journey.

> *"Once the pain goes away, the positive memories come back. Laughter has kept me going, along with my daughter Julie. Bob has his own table and a picture of him lies on top along with a candle and a little sign saying 'Bobbleberry', which was from the grandchildren and great-grandchildren. They called him 'Bobbleberry'. This makes us laugh and brings back pleasant memories of Bob and the things he said. We talk about him all the time. Every evening, Julie and I raise a glass to Bob and we say, 'Remember Bob!'"*
> *Edna*

SUMMARY

The dementia journey will be different for everyone. The reactions to the challenges can vary by intensity, but also by how people respond to each stage. Trying to maintain wellbeing for you and your loved one throughout the transitions will depend on a delicate balance of perceived need, risk and likelihood of resolution at each part of the journey. Explore options for formal systems of support in advance of needing them from formal carers, respite options, care homes and end-of-life care. You will always be connected to your loved one, albeit in a different way and with the involvement of others.

KEY POINTS TO REMEMBER

- There will be different options for formal care to support your loved one, depending on your personal circumstances. It is important to explore these.
- Consider your needs alongside your loved one's needs when considering formal care arrangements.
- It is normal for settling your loved one into a care home to bring up many feelings, so self-care remains just as important.
- As your loved one approaches the end of their life remember that your care and connection sustained them through this journey. As always, self-care is critical at this stage.

FINAL WORDS

Throughout the book, we have focused on what you can do to support your loved one's changing needs, alongside looking after yourself. There is so much that can be done to improve the quality of life for you both. How far do you think you have come in changing your mind about dementia since you began reading? It is OK to feel unsure. It would be almost impossible to take on everything we have discussed in one reading, so please keep going back to the relevant chapters.

The principles of person-centred care and drawing on your values offer a way to appreciate and care for your loved one, through the good times and the bad. Focus on what is within your control and set meaningful goals using the strategies outlined regarding quality of life, self-care, communication, and your own reactions and responses. These ideas and strategies will take practice so whenever you falter, remind yourself why you are doing this and watch out for your inner critic when challenges arise; please do not give up. These strategies are designed to be flexible and there is no one right way. Celebrate the exceptions and successes and learn to trust your instincts and creativity. Being in the moment is precious – make the most of now. Nurture your skills of self-compassion. And remember, do not try to do this alone. Reach out to others and sustain supportive connections to keep you going. It is within everyone's control to challenge the stigma and tell a different story of dementia.

APPENDICES

HOW TO PREPARE AN ADVANCE DIRECTIVE

ADVANCE DECISIONS – A LIVING WILL

This sets out the situations in which a person may want to refuse medical treatment should they lack the mental capacity to make or communicate that decision in the future. This is to assist decisions about the person's diagnosis and prognosis, which will be made by the doctor in charge of care. Here are the key features of an advance decision:

- **Personal details:** Full name, address, date of birth, medical number – public or private services, health insurance details
- **Doctor's details:** Surgery, contacts, other specialties
- **Who the advance decision has been discussed with:** Names and contact details

- **Refusal of treatment:** This should apply when life is at risk or it is shortened by it. This includes dementia of any type, brain injury, diseases of the central nervous system, terminal illness or the refusal of treatment in other situations. State which of these diagnoses will entail refusal of treatment.
- **Pain relief:** Outline preferences and whether all means can be used
- **Organ donation:** Outline preferences
- **Advance Statement:** Explains why this advance decision exists and what is important to the person in relation to health, care and quality of life
- **Who are the people the person would like to be involved in their care?** Names and give contact details
- **Details of Lasting Power of Attorney for Health, Welfare and Finances:** Name the registered attorneys
- **Signature**
- **Witness details of the signature**
- **Review dates of the document:** Keep a list of the review dates at the back of the document, which will be an indication that the contents truly and accurately reflect the person's wishes.

Based on Compassion in Dying's template[34]

COMMON BEHAVIOURS THAT CHALLENGE

Direct Forms of Behaviour	Indirect Forms of Behaviour
Hitting	Repetitive noise
Kicking	Repetitive questions
Grabbing	Making strange noises
Pushing	Constant requests for help
Nipping	Eating/drinking excessively
Scratching	Over-activity
Biting	Pacing
Spitting	General agitation
Choking	Following others/trailing
Hair pulling	Inappropriate exposure of parts of body
Tripping	Masturbating in public areas
Throwing objects	Urinating in inappropriate places
Stick prodding	Smearing faeces
Stabbing	Handling things inappropriately
Swearing	Dismantling objects
Screaming	Hoarding things
Shouting	Hiding items
Physical sexual assault	Falling intentionally
Verbal sexual advances	Ingesting inappropriate substances
Acts of self-harm	Non-compliance with taking medications

Adapted from James (2011)

DELIRIUM CHECKLIST

Getting to Know Delirium	
Causes	**Risk Factors**
• Pain • Infection • Constipation • Dehydration • Reaction to medication and withdrawal from it	• Dementia – people with dementia are five times more likely to have delirium • Poor vision or hearing problems • Disorientation • Dehydration • Constipation • Poor nutrition • Urine catheters (increased risk of infection) • Illness • Immobility and falls • Polypharmacy – taking lots of medications

Recognizing Signs and Symptoms of Delirium

- Have you noticed a sudden change in your loved one?

- Do they seem to have been more confused than usual over the last few hours or days?

- Does the confusion fluctuate during the day? What are morning, evening and night times like? When are they at their best? Are they more confused at night?

- Do they seem to have more difficulty than usual concentrating?

- Do they find it hard to follow a conversation or are they easily distracted?

- Do they seem to be jumping from one topic to another?

- Does their thinking seem more disorganized than usual?

- Is your loved one having unusual experiences? Hearing or seeing things that are not real? Have they unusual beliefs about what is going on around them?

- Does your loved one seem more agitated or more sleepy than usual?

- Are there changes in sleep patterns?

TROUBLESHOOTING DEMENTIA, DELIRIUM AND DEPRESSION: UNDERSTANDING THE SIMILARITIES AND DIFFERENCES

If you see agitated behaviour, you are encouraged to think about the commonalities that delirium, dementia and depression have, but also their differences. Delirium can be difficult to tell apart from other common problems – dementia and depression, in this case. It's especially tricky if someone has delirium in addition to dementia or depression, but this is very common. This table gives some useful pointers for telling them apart.

	Delirium	Dementia	Depression
Onset	Sudden (hours/days)	Usually gradual (months/years)	Gradual (weeks/months)
Alertness	Fluctuates	Generally normal	Generally normal
Attention	Fluctuates – poor focus and distractible	Generally normal	Some difficulty concentrating, distractible
Sleep	Change in sleeping pattern (often more confused at night)	Can be disturbed/ night-time wandering and confusion possible	Early-morning wakening, excessive sleeping
Thinking	Disorganized – jumping from one idea to another	Poor problem-solving, poor judgement, language problems	Slower, negative thinking e.g., hopelessness, despair, self-criticism
Perception	Illusions, delusions and hallucinations	Generally normal	Generally normal

ACKNOWLEDGEMENTS

Thank you to our editor Beth Bishop, for asking us to write this book. It has been an honour to share our understandings and hopefully improve the wellbeing of others going through this journey. Thank you for your guidance, support, commitment and responsiveness along the way.

Our deepest gratitude to family members, friends and colleagues who have sustained our commitment to this book; we are very grateful to all of you for sharing your personal and professional insights. In particular we would like to thank Dr Navi Nagra, Dr Line Sagfors, Jane Sweetman, Catriona McCarthy, Ruth Lisk, Eoin Hamill, Kathleen McCarthy, Peter Booth, Sharon Leen, Mary McCarthy, Paul Scannell, Bea Bellec, Simon Widlo, Lesley Smith, Victor Bellec, Aisling Ryan, Claire Smith, Dr Juliette Brown, Agnes Sagfors and Dr Kate Mahony. Thank you for taking the time to read and re-read the drafts that formed this book. All of you have left your mark.

ENDNOTES

1. Kitwood, 1997
2. Vernooij-Dassen & Moniz-Cook, 2016
3. Burnham, 1993; 2008
4. Brooker, 2007
5. Epictetus, 1995
6. Pausch & Zaslow, 2008
7. Mosconi, 2020
8. Rahman et al 2020
9. Whitehouse, 2008
10. Norton, 2014
11. Harris, 2008
12. Harris, 2008
13. Harris, 2008
14. Taylor, 2007
15. White & Epston,1990
16. Ncube, p. 7, 2006
17. Carrillo, 2016

18. Harris, 2011
19. Harris, 2019
20. Gilbert, 2010
21. Sedgewick, 2014
22. Killick & Allan, 2008
23. Ellis & Astell, 2008
24. Caldwell, 2005
25. Moniz-Cook et al., 2012
26. Cohen-Mansfield, 2000
27. James, 2011
28. Moniz-Cook & James, 2017
29. James & Hope, 2013
30. Kitwood, 1997
31. Ncube-Mlilo, 2013
32. Ncube, 2006
33. Byock, 2014
34. compassionindying.org.uk/library/advance-decision-pack/

REFERENCES

Alzheimer's Association (2020). '2020 Alzheimer's disease facts and figures'. *Alzheimer's & Dementia: The Journal of the Alzheimer's Association*, 16, 3, 391–460. Available online: www.alz.org/media/Documents/alzheimers-facts-and-figures.pdf

Alzheimer's Disease International (2019). 'World Alzheimer Report, 2019: Attitudes to Dementia'. Available online: www.alz.co.uk/research/world-report-2019

Brooker, D. (2007). *Person-centred Dementia Care. Making Services Better.* London and Philadelphia: Jessica Kingsley Publishing

Bryden, C. (2005). *Dancing with Dementia: My Story of Living Positively with Dementia.* London and Philadelphia: Jessica Kingsley Publishing

Burnham, J. (1993). 'Systemic supervision: The evolution of reflexivity in the context of the supervisory relationship'. *Human Systems*, 4, 349–381.

Burnham, J., Alvis Palma, D., and Whitehouse, L. (2008). 'Learning as a context for differences and differences as a context for learning' *Journal of Family Therapy*, 30, 529–542.

Byock, I. (2014). *The Four Things that Matter Most – 10th Anniversary Edition: A Book About Living.* New York: Atria Books

Caldwell, P. (2005). *Finding You Finding Me: Using Intensive Interaction to get in touch with people whose severe learning disabilities are combined with autistic spectrum disorder.* London: Jessica Kingsley Publishing

Carrillo, M. (2016). 'Why Does Alzheimer's Disease Affect More Women Than Men? New Alzheimer's Association Grant Will Help Researchers Explore That Question'. *Alz Blog.* Available online: www.alz.org/blog/alz/february_2016/why_does_alzheimer_s_disease_affect_more_women_tha

Cohen-Mansfield, J. (2000). 'Use of patient characteristics to determine non-pharmacologic interventions for behavioural and psychological symptoms of dementia'. *International Psychogeriatrics*, 12 (suppl. 1), 373–380.

Ellis, M.P., and Astell, A.J. (2008). 'Promoting communication with people with severe dementia' in S. Zeedyk (Ed) *Techniques for*

Promoting Social Engagement in Individuals with Communicative Impairments. London: Jessica Kingsley Publishing

Epictetus (1995). *A Manual for Living (Little Books of Wisdom).* San Francisco: Harper

Gilbert, P. (2010). *Compassion Focused Therapy: The CBT Distinctive Features Series.* London, UK: Routledge. www.compassionatemind.co.uk

Harris, R. (2008). *The Happiness Trap. Based on ACT: A revolutionary mindfulness-based programme for overcoming stress, anxiety and depression.* London: Robinson. www.thehappinesstrap.com

Harris, R. (2012). *The Reality Slap. How to find fulfilment when life hurts.* London: Robinson. www.actmindfully.com.au

Harris, R. (2019). *ACT Made Simple: the Extra Bits.* [eBook] Available at: ACT-made-simple-The-Extra-Bits-Russ-Harris-May-2019-version2.pdf

James, I. (2011). *Understanding Behaviour in Dementia that Challenges: A Guide to Assessment and Treatment.* London: Jessica Kingsley Publishing

James, I. and Hope, A. (2013). 'Relevance of emotions and beliefs in the treatment of behaviors that challenge in dementia patients'. *Neurodegenerative Disease Management*, 3, 575–588.

Kabat-Zinn, J. (2013). *Full Catastrophe Living, Revised Edition: How to cope with stress, pain and illness using mindfulness meditation.* London: Piatkus

Killick, J., and Allan, K. (2008). *Communication and the Care of People with Dementia*, 3rd edn, Maidenhead: Open University Press

Kitwood, T. (1997). *Dementia Reconsidered: The Person Comes First.* Croydon: Open University Press

Moniz-Cook E.D., Swift, K., James, I., Malouf, R., De Vugt, M. and Verhey, F. (2012). 'Functional analysis-based interventions for challenging behaviour in dementia'. *Cochrane Database System Review*, 2.

Moniz-Cook, E., and James, I. (2017). '"Behaviour that challenges" in dementia care: An update of psychological approaches for home and care home settings'. *FPOP Bulletin*, 140, 43–49.

Mosconi, L. (2020). *The XX Brain: The Groundbreaking Science Empowering Women to Prevent Dementia,* London: Allen & Unwin

Ncube, N. (2006). 'The tree of life project. Using narrative ideas in work with vulnerable children in southern Africa'. *International Journal of Narrative Therapy & Community Work*, 2006(1), 3–16.

Ncube-Mlilo, N. (2013). 'Narratives in the suitcase'. Video Presentation. Available online: dulwichcentre.com.au/narratives-in-the-suitcase-by-ncazelo-ncube-mlilo

Norton S, Matthews FE, Barnes DE, Yaffe K, Brayne C. (2014). 'Potential for primary prevention of Alzheimer's disease: an analysis of population-based data'. *Lancet Neurol.* 13 (8) 788-94.

Pausch, R., and Zaslow, J. (2008). *The Last Lecture.* New York: Hyperion

Power, G.A. (2014). *Dementia Beyond Disease: Enhancing Well-Being, First Edition.* New York: Health Professions Press

Rahman A., Schelbaum E., Hoffman K., Diaz I., Hristov H., Andrews R., et al. (2020). 'Sex-driven modifiers of Alzheimer risk: A multimodality brain imaging study'. **Neurology**, 95 (2) 166–178.

Sedgewick, R. (2014). 'Communicating effectively with a person living with a dementia'. *Belfast Health and Social Care Trust.* Available online: www.publichealth.hscni.net/sites/default/files/dementia%20booklet_07_16%20%285%29.pdf

Taylor, R. (2007). *Alzheimer's from the Inside Out.* New York: Health Professions Press

Vernooij-Dassen, M. and Moniz-Cook, E. (2016). 'Person-centred dementia care: moving beyond caregiving'. *Aging & Mental Health*, 20:7, 667–668.

White, M. (1988/9). 'The externalizing of the problem and the re-authoring of lives and relationships' in M. White (Ed.), *Selected Papers (pp. 5-28).* Adelaide, Australia: Dulwich Centre Publications

White, M., and Epston, D. (1990). *Narrative Means to Therapeutic Ends.* New York: W. W. Norton

Whitehouse, P.J. (2008). *The Myth of Alzheimer's. What you aren't being told about today's most dreaded diagnosis.* New York: St Martin's Griffin

World Health Organization [WHO] (2020). *Dementia: Key Facts.* Available online: www.who.int/news-room/fact-sheets/detail/dementia

USEFUL RESOURCES

UK & EUROPE

Dementia UK provides specialist dementia support for families through their Admiral Nurse service: www.dementiauk.org

Compassion in Dying, a UK charity, encourages talking about and planning for end of life and dying with dignity: compassionindying.org.uk/choose-a-way-to-make-an-advance-decision-living-will

Alzheimer's Society, a UK care and research charity, provides an array of information, publications and support: www.alzheimers.org.uk

Useful resources for self-care are available from Paul Gilbert at the Compassionate Mind Foundation: www.compassionatemind.co.uk

Russ Harris' website has information on values and self-care: www.actmindfully.come.au/free-stuff

'Dementia animations' are a product of collaboration between Cumbria, Northumberland, Tyne and Wear NHS Foundation Trust (authored by Ian Andrew James) and the British Psychological Society, Division of Clinical Psychology, Faculty of the Psychology of Older People – FPOP. These include:

- "Memory in Dementia" (youtu.be/aSx5sUVBcCE)
- "Sensory changes in Dementia" (youtu.be/KHUijkp-kj)
- "Needs in Dementia" (youtu.be/R0C2ug7AbT)

Rare Dementia Support is a UK-based service led by the UCL Dementia Research Centre (DRC) who aim to empower, guide and inform people living with a rare dementia diagnosis and those who care about them: www.raredementiasupport.org

YoungDementia UK, part of Dementia UK, provide advice and support for people affected by young onset dementia: www.youngdementiauk.org

Alzheimer Europe is a non-profit non-governmental organization (NGO) aiming to provide a voice to people with dementia and their carers, make dementia a European priority, promote a rights-based approach to dementia, support dementia research and strengthen the European dementia movement. www.alzheimer-europe.org

UNITED STATES

Alzheimer's Association, an American voluntary health organization in Alzheimer's care, support and research: www.alz.org

Alzheimer's Society of Canada is a registered charity providing advice, support, collaboration and research for the benefit of people living with dementia in Canada: alzheimer.ca

AFRICA

DementiaSA is a South African Non-Profit Organization (NPO) that assists families, communities and health professionals who have limited access to private healthcare, to live with dementia or care for those with dementia: www.dementiasa.org

Africa Dementia Service is an organization promoting awareness of dementia across Africa: africadementiaservices.com

AUSTRALASIA

Dementia Australia, a non-profit charity, provide excellent help sheets and resources: www.dementia.org.au/information

Dementia New Zealand and its regional affiliates aim to be by the side of individuals, families, networks and communities to ensure anyone affected by dementia has the freedom and confidence to make the most of every day: dementia.nz

SOUTH ASIA

Meri Yaadain – recognizing dementia within South Asian communities – language leaflets and audio clips in South Asian languages: www.meriyaadain.co.uk

Dementia Care Notes India is a website that draws together supports and organizations for people with dementia in India: dementiacarenotes.in/resources/india

Triggerhub.Org is one of the most elite and scientifically proven forms of mental health intervention

Trigger Publishing is the leading independent mental health and wellbeing publisher in the UK and US. Clinical and scientific research conducted by assistant professor Dr Kristin Kosyluk and her highly acclaimed team in the Department of Mental Health Law & Policy at the University of South Florida (USF), as well as complementary research by her peers across the US, has independently verified the power of lived experience as a core component in achieving mental health prosperity. Specifically, the lived experiences contained within our bibliotherapeutic books are intrinsic elements in reducing stigma, making those with poor mental health feel less alone, providing the privacy they need to heal, ensuring they know the essential steps to kick-start their own journeys to recovery, and providing hope and inspiration when they need it most.

Delivered through TriggerHub, our unique online portal and accompanying smartphone app, we make our library of bibliotherapeutic titles and other vital resources accessible to individuals and organizations anywhere, at any time and with complete privacy, a crucial element of recovery. As such, TriggerHub is the primary recommendation across the UK and US for the delivery of lived experiences.

At Trigger Publishing and TriggerHub, we proudly lead the way in making the unseen become seen. We are dedicated to humanizing mental health, breaking stigma and challenging outdated societal values to create real action and impact. Find out more about our world-leading work with lived experience and bibliotherapy via triggerhub. org, or by joining us on:

🐦 @triggerhub_

f @triggerhub.org

📷 @triggerhub_

9 781837 962600